Bircher-Benner Diet Books

Manual for patients with gastrointestinal conditions

Dietary instructions
for days of health and illness,
with recipes,
detailed advice
and a sophisticated treatment plan
from a medical centre for
state-of-the-art healing.

Dr. med. Andres Bircher
Editor: Irène Hagmann

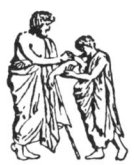

EDITION BIRCHER-BENNER
CH-8784 BRAUNWALD

Bircher-Benner manuals

1. Manual for patients with multiple sclerosis and degenerative nervous diseases
2. Manual for patients with liver and gallbladder conditions
3. Manual for families and children
4. Manual of fresh juices, raw vegetables and fruit dishes
5. Manual for improvement of the immune system and against susceptibility to infection
6. Manual for mountaineers and athletes
7. Manual for diabetics
8. Manual for support and preventive therapy for lung diseases
9. Enjoy food without table salt
10. Manual for patients with rheumatism and arthritis
11. Manual for men with prostate conditions
12. Manual for patients with kidney and bladder conditions
13. Manual for venous diseases
14. Manual for patients with gastrointestinal conditions
15. Manual for nutrition during pregnancy and lactation
16. Manual for gynaecological problems and menopause
17. Manual for the prevention of cancer and accompanying therapies
18. Manual for headache and migraine
19. Manual for patients with hypertension, cardiovascular disease and arteriosclerosis
20. Manual for overcoming anxiety and depression
21. Manual for patients with skin diseases or sensitive skin
22. Manual for persons suffering from stress
23. Manual for persons suffering from allergies
24. Manual for prevention of dementia and Alzheimer's disease
25. Manual for internal treatment of eye problems
26. Manual for treatment of weight problems, overweight, and anorexia

These manuals are the results of global research, the development of the art and science of medicine across more than a century and the experience of the renowned Bircher-Benner Klinik. The reader will feel the helpful support of the well-informed physician at every step of the way.

24th edition fully revised 2015. Translated from the original German.

All rights reserved, including the right of reproduction in excerpts, photomechanical reproduction or translation
info@bircher-benner.com   www.bircher-benner.com

Book orders: edition@bircher-benner.com
© Copyright Edition Bircher-Benner, CH 8784 Braunwald
® The trademarks Bircher and Bircher-Benner are protected worldwide
Printed in Germany

The suggestions in this book have been carefully reviewed by the authors and the publisher. However, we cannot assume any guarantee.
The authors and the publishers hereby disclaim all liability for personal injury, property damage and all types of financial loss.

Cover design: Kösel Media GmbH, Krugzell
Overall production: Kösel, Krugzell

Table of Contents

Preface 7

Structure of the Digestive Tract 8
    The Mouth 8
    The Oesophagus 8
    The Stomach 9
    The Duodenum 9
    The Pancreas 9
    The Jejunum 10
    The Ileum 11
    The Enterohepatic Circulation 11
    The Colon 11
    The Immune System of the Intestine 12
    The Intestinal Flora 12
    Regulation of the Digestive System 13
    Hormonal Regulation of Digestion 13

Diseases of the Oesophagus 15
    Swallowing Problems 15
    Reflux and Diaphragmatic Hernia 15
    Barrett Oesophagus (endobrachyoesophagus) 15
    Therapy of Reflux and Barrett Syndrome 15
    Cancer of the Oesophagus (Oesophageal Carcinoma) 16

Diseases of the Stomach 17
    Gastritis 17
    The Over-Acidic Stomach (Chronic Gastritis) 17
    The Acid-Deficient, Slack Stomach 17
    Colonisation of the Stomach by *Helicobacter Pylori* 18

Stomach Cancer	18
Diseases of the Pancreas	**20**
Acute Pancreatitis	20
Chronic Pancreatitis	20
Pancreatic Cancer (Pancreatic Carcinoma)	20
Failure of the Pancreas (Pancreas Insufficiency)	20
Diseases of the Intestine	**21**
Duodenal Ulcer (Ulcus duodeni)	21
Intestinal Catarrh (Enteritis, Colitis, Fermentation, Rot)	21
Constipation and Diarrhoea	22
Intestinal Putrefaction and Fermentation, Bacterial Miscolonization	23
Miscolonization of the Small Intestine	24
Intestinal Putrefaction	24
Therapy of Bacterial Miscolonization	24
Appendicitis	25
Meteorism	26
Irritable Bowel Syndrome	27
Coeliac Disease (Herter's Disease)	28
Lactose Intolerance	31
Fructose Intolerance	32
Histamine Intolerance	33
The Problem of Food Allergy	34
Crohn's disease	34
Colitis Ulcerosa	39
Diverticular Disease (Diverticulosis)	42
Cancer of the Large Intestine (Colon Carcinoma)	43
The Effect of Food on the Digestive Tract	**47**
Two types of food energy	47
General Guidelines for Treatment of Intestinal Diseases	**49**
The Raw Apple Diet (Especially in Case of Diarrhoea)	49
The Raw Food Diet	49

The Sour Milk Diet	50
Notes on Choice of Foods	50
Diet Types	**52**
Diet I Tea Fasting	52
Diet II Juices	52
A. For Acute Diarrhoea	52
B. For Overly Acidic Stomach, Ulcers	54
C. For Acid-Deficient Stomach	55
Diet III Pureed Food (Mash)	56
Diet IV Bland Healing Diet	58
Diet V Protective Healing Diet	59
Permanent Diet for Frequent Constipation	59
The Recipes	**61**
Juices	61
Healthful Teas	62
Muesli	63
Raw vegetables and salads	65
Salad dressings	66
Suggestions for dressings to go with the salads and raw vegetables	69
Milk Types	70
Butter, vegetable fats and oils – gentle cooking and steaming/sautéing	70
Gentle cooking and steaming/sautéing	71
Soups	71
Vegetables	74
Salads of cooked vegetables	80
Potato Dishes	82
Cereal Dishes	84
Sauces	87
Sandwiches	89
Desserts	90
Suggestion for menus Sorted according to Different Consistancy Types	**94**
Summary of the Foods for the Healing Diet for Digestive Problems*	**98**

Indications for General Applications for Gastrointestinal Disease 100
    Baths 100
        Kuhne's friction hip bath 100
        Alternating foot bath 100
        Cold half-bath *(according to Winternitz, Kuhne, Kneipp)* 100
    Washes 101
        Cold abdominal wash 101
        Full wash 101
        Body wash 101
        Lower abdominal wash 101
        Abdominal wash 101
    Cold gushes (Kneipp, Winternitz) 101
        Thigh gush 101
        The abdominal gush according to Winternitz 102
    Compresses 102
        Kuhne and Priessnitz body compresses 102
    Compresses and applications 102
        Kneipp steam compress 102
    Massages 103
        Belly massage (Winternitz method) 103

Diet Table for Patients with Gastrointestinal Diseases 104

List of Recipes 107

Notes 108

Index 113

Preface

We need the stomach and intestine not only for ingesting food and drink, but also to form a comprehensive, well developed, graduated pre-mechanism of our organism in its self-defence against the environmental influences that would make it ill. The entire digestive tract houses an inner external world that penetrates our body and exposes it to any number of mechanical, chemical and microbial stimuli and influences against which it must isolate and defend itself. The structure – comprising the cellular and biochemical functions of the gastrointestinal tract – is ingenuously designed to meet the requirements of continuous differentiation between what is foreign and its own, between the useful (vital) and harmful (destructive) input penetrating it. The digestive tract is a masterpiece of nature. The symbiosis (i.e. interaction) of our intestine with the approx. 20 trillion germs of our intestinal flora, a complex ecosystem without which we could not survive, has developed over the course of millions of years. As long as our digestive system is in good condition and functional, we are protected from any adverse effects due to defects and errors in our nutrition. However, if the stomach and intestine become weakened or ill, they can cause general sickliness, since the entire biological system will slowly lose its complex, dynamic balance. *Therefore the persons suffering from gastrointestinal problems must be extremely careful in their choice of nutrition. They must recover the health of their intestinal milieu as quickly as possible, if they are to avoid suffering from general degenerative diseases in subsequent years.* An energetically and materially healthful nutrition, as well as a healthy biochemical and microbial milieu in the digestive tract, are what the entire complex system of our metabolism depends on. Likewise, the maintenance of our basic regulation, and the entire energy and information flow in the biological system of our bodies. The quality of our food determines our fate: regeneration or degeneration, illness or health.

This series of manuals explains how to prevent and heal the chronic diseases that occur with increasing frequency (and increasingly early) in life. Practical aids include preventive and healing dietary instructions, as well as measures, which support and control the self-healing efforts of our organism. Explanations and instructions are based on scientific insights which are still in evidence.
Our dietary instructions have been refined through decades of experience. They prove to be extremely efficient. Here we show clearly and in an easily comprehensible manner how to proceed to heal gastrointestinal diseases in practice. Whatever the problem, we would nevertheless recommend close cooperation with your attending physician, for whom this book will be a great help in treating his or her patients.

Braunwald, 22. January 2014
Dr. med. Andres Bircher

Structure of the Digestive Tract

The Mouth

The first place to look for maintaining health is the mouth, which is all too easily forgotten in this context. The mouth is naturally equipped to fulfil a number of important tasks in the ingestion of nutrients: mash-like chopping, salivation for pre-digestion, and inspection of food for wholesomeness, aided by the senses of touch, temperature and taste of the tongue and smell mediated by the choanae. Viewed in evolutionary terms, human dentition is equipped only with incisors and molars for eating fruits, plants and grains. Fangs and powerful premolars, present in dogs, cats and predators and used to tear and cut meat, are missing in humans. Six salivary glands produce daily about one litre of saliva, rich in amylase, a first digestive enzyme for pre-digestion of starch. The tongue can recognise sugar, salt, bitter substances and acids. Any finer sense of taste is ensured by the sensory cells of the nose, which perceive smell through the choanae, internal nostrils found at the back of the throat. The throat develops over the course of life and may be dulled or refined. The act of swallowing can be triggered voluntarily only at the beginning; after the epiglottis has closed, swallowing becomes involuntary, a large wave-like motion of the throat that will pass into the peristaltic waves of the oesophagus.

The appearance, smell and taste of food put the entire digestive system into motion, change the intestinal milieu – peristalsis and appetitive behaviour – and prepare it in a suitable direction. Careful chewing is particularly important. If chewing is partially prevented (e.g. because of a lack of ability of the teeth to chew), digestive impairment will be the rule. Hunger is something very different from appetite. There are actually two kinds of appetite. The mouth, sense of taste and smell engage spontaneously. Always 'ask' your stomach if it likes the food it is receiving and if it will tolerate it, and then listen to what your metabolism 'says' about it.

The oral cavity is lined with flat cell layers (multi-layered squamous epithelium) and handles injury surprisingly well. Frequent injury and burns from excessively hot or spicy foods, or overly frequent use of alcohol or tobacco, may lead to cell mutation causing very dangerous oral cancer. Hot food, alcoholic drinks and tobacco must be avoided.

The Oesophagus

Located behind the larynx and trachea, the oesophagus connects the throat to the entrance of the stomach. Equipped with layers of strong muscle, the oesophagus transports food swallowed through a gap in the diaphragm and down into the stomach. In a healthy person, the oesophagus is protected from returning stomach content and acid by a strong fold of the stomach (cardia). The multi-layered plate-like cell layers (squamous epithelium) protect the oesophagus from injury and burns from excessively hot or spicey food. The oesophagus is innervated by branches of the vagus nerve and from spinal cord segments that are reflectorily connected to the heart. Therefore swallowing problems or belching into the oesophagus may appear as heart pain.

The Stomach

Placed from the left to the right under the diaphragm, the left half of the stomach (fundus) takes in food. During this stage, this part will slacken to prevent pressure. In the middle of the stomach, there is the pacemaker centre where peristaltic waves that move the stomach content in the direction of the exit porter (pylorus) are emitted. The pylorus remains closed until the food is sufficiently digested to be supplied to the small intestine. Endocrine cells of the stomach wall produce gastrin, a hormone that increases the peristaltic waves and the excretion of acid and enzyme. The mucosa of the stomach is highly active; its cells are quickly replaced. Parietal cells of the stomach produce hydrochloric acid, and goblet cells produce gastric mucus to protect the stomach wall. Every day, 1–4 litres of gastric juice are produced to strongly acidify the chyme and add the stomach enzyme pepsin that breaks down the proteins into amino acids. Food intake promotes the formation of acidic gastric juice via reflexes of our vegetative nervous system. The appearance, smell or thought of food is enough to trigger this. If even very small amounts of food enter the lower part of the stomach (antrum pylori), the stomach wall will stimulate additional production of acidic gastric juice via the hormone gastrin. *Overly frequent eating or snacking will cause massive acidification of the stomach and reflux because of continuous overextension of the stomach fundus. The continuous slackening of the stomach fundus will cause the stomach entrance to leak, thereby allowing acidic stomach content to enter the oesophagus.* Breaks of at least four hours are needed to keep the stomach regulation healthy.

If stomach content is too acidic (pH below 1.5–3), the stomach will automatically switch off acid production. When the stomach content has emptied into the small intestine, the small intestine will excrete the hormones secretin and GIP, which also inhibit the stomach. A healthy stomach will prepare its contents carefully before emptying them into the small intestine. These ingenious regulation processes are very sensitive. They can be easily impaired by the wrong lifestyle and poor nutrition, by addictive behaviour and stress, and by stimulants such as coffee and alcohol, roasted substances and nicotine, until severe illness results.

The Duodenum

To the right, below the liver, the duodenum is situated as an S-shaped loop in front of the back muscles. It is the first part of the small intestine that conveys the food to the left into the long jejunum. In addition to emitting the hormone secretin, which inhibits the gastric juice production once filled with food from the stomach, the duodenum receives secretions from the pancreas mixed with gall from the liver. The pancreas secretion buffers the stomach acid with its high content of sodium bicarbonate. The wall cells of the duodenum activate the digestive enzymes of the pancreas. The gall from the liver binds to fatty substances and splits them up into glycerine and free fatty acids during their passage through the small intestine.

The Pancreas

The pancreas is our largest digestive gland. Behind the stomach, embedded into the loop of the duodenum, it twists around the spleen vein like an eel. At its centre is the main duct of the gland (ductus pancreaticus). Before it merges into the duodenum in the 'head' of the pancreas, it absorbs the large bile duct (ductus choledochus). Every day the pancreas produces 1 to 2 litres of alkaline digestive juice, rich in sodium bicarbonate and preliminary stages of the protein-splitting digestive enzymes trypsin and chymotrypsin, the starch-splitting amylasis and the fat-splitting lipase, to name only the most important ones. These pre-stages are inactive, so that the pancreas will not digest itself. Excreted into the small intestine, the pancreatic enzymes are activated by messenger substances at slightly alkaline pH values, and begin their digestive work. The small intestine's hormone secretin strongly stimulates the pancreas when the bolus (food pulp) arrives, as does the hormone cholecystokinin, which also signals the gall bladder to empty itself when fatty substances enter the duodenum. If our senses are focused on food or if we are stressed or preoccupied, the pancreas will also be overstimulated via the vagus nerve. If the bolus (food pulp) of the small intestine already contains enough protein-digesting trypsin, the pancreas will be inhibited in order to prevent self-digestion.

There is also the hormonal activity of the pancreas (endocrine pancreas), since this organ is shot through with innumerable cell islands (the islet cells). If the glucose sugar level in the blood increases because sugar substances or starch have been eaten, the β-cells of these islets release the hormone insulin. Only the effect of this hormone in all cell membranes of the body permits glucose to enter the cells and be used in the mitochondria, the 'power plants' of our cells. If the blood sugar level drops too far, the α-cells of these islets will release the hormone glucagon. Glucagon raises the glucose level in the blood by stimulating the degradation of starch (glycogen out) in the liver into glucose and promotes its new production from catabolites. The hormone glucagon from the pancreas thus ensures sufficient supply of all cells by means of sugar between meals. In emergency situations, at even higher energy demand, the adrenal hormones adrenaline and cortisol will come into play to ensure sugar supply. Once sufficient glucose and arginine have entered the cells after eating, the δ-cells of the islets produce the hormone somatomedin, which inhibits the release of insulin.

These regulatory processes are very sensitive to impairment of the stomach and small intestine, mental stress, unnatural nutrition, overly frequent meals, drugs and stimulants. Therefore the pancreas also requires long breaks between the meals or food intake.

The Jejunum

This longest part of the small intestine is 3–6 metres long, with muscle layers for peristalsis and a very densely constructed inner layer of mucosa. It is supplied with strong blood vessels through the peritoneum. The veins of the small and large intestine belong to the portal vein system and route the blood to the liver. The lipids are split up by the bile acids into glycerine, free fatty acids and other fat fragments. The intestinal cells 'pack' the lipids into the smallest fat droplets (chylomicrons) as an emulsion and pass them on to the lymphatic system of the intestine. From there they enter the venous blood through the main lymphatic vessel, where the lipids are bound to protein substances (lipoproteins) by enzymes and the remaining fatty acids are split off to serve as nutrients for the muscle cells.

The surface of the small intestine is so much enlarged by dense folds, bulges and dents (similar to a coral reef) that it reaches a total of approx. 200 m^2. The cells of the mucosa of the small intestine are subject to enormous stress every day, requiring them to be replaced by new, young cells every 3–4 days. Goblet cells produce a thick mucus layer that covers the entire intestinal mucosa. The mucus is penetrated by IgA antibodies that belong to everything our intestine knows and has learned to tolerate as harmless – like an immunology memory. The healthy intestinal mucosa carefully seals our body against the intestinal content that belongs to the outside world, and compatible nutrients, subject to strict control, pass only through the cells. In an irritated intestinal wall, the mucus layer of the small intestine is deficient. Additionally, the connection points between the cells ('tight junctions') begin to leak so that nutrients, foreign substances and toxins can pass partially uncontrolled through the diseased intestinal wall. The immune system reacts to them with allergic immune reactions. The healthy small intestine has a resting peristalsis (slow waves) that is very important for an orderly digestive process. It produces more than 2 litres of mucus and digestive juices every day. Just like the large intestine, its inner layer is covered by a specific dense bacterial "lawn" without which we would be unable to survive. The intestinal content is light in colour and slightly acidic in the case of healthful nutrition and in breastfed infants.

The Ileum

This is the last, short section of the small intestine before it merges with the large intestine. In this part of the intestine, the bound (conjugated) bile acids are absorbed and returned via the portal vein to the liver for recycling. Another special feature of the ileum is resorption of vitamin B_{12} (cobalamin). For this, the ileum mucosa requires the 'intrinsic factor' from healthy stomach mucosa.

The Enterohepatic Circulation

The nutrients from the intestine are supplied to the liver via the portal vein system and the resorbed lipids are passed on to the metabolism via the lymphatic system in the form of very fine fat droplets (chylomicrons). In the liver cells, the food is used efficiently for the metabolism and toxins are carefully removed.

Nutrients supplied in senseless excess will overburden the liver. Everything that its cells cannot handle will be returned to the small intestine via the gall, stressing it again through this second digestive cycle. The small intestine then returns the entire superfluous supply to the liver through the portal vein system, which in turn endeavours to process it. Thus nutrients and toxins move in the enterohepatic circulation[1] between the intestine and liver until the entire excessive supply can be processed. The excessive stress on the enterohepatic circulation becomes evident in great fatigue experienced after meals, extended fatigue crises and haemorrhoids. This symptom is the alarm signal of a dangerous overburdening of the metabolism due to excessive and poor nutrition and is widespread today. See our Manual no. 2 for patients with Liver and Gall Bladder Conditions, in which the consequences of this overburdening and the dietary path for healing it are described.

The Colon

This last part of the intestine is about 1.3 m long and comprises the following: a blind start (caecum with appendix), which merges with the small intestine; the ascending colon; the transcending colon; and the descending colon, which leads to the rectum via an S-shaped (sigma) loop. There are deep regular folds. The colon has three main tasks: re-absorption of water, so that the daily stool mass (chymus) of the small intestine is thickened from 500–1500 ml to 100–200 ml; reabsorption of salt particles (electrolytes) from the stool to prevent salt loss; and storage of the stool masses until discharge is possible. The ascending large intestine and the rectum serve as storage. At the end of the caecum is the appendix, a very narrow portion of intestine. Similar to the tonsils in the oral cavity, it is needed for immune defence as a kind of intestinal tonsil. From the expanded section (rectal ampulla), the rectum crosses the sphincter muscle of the anus before transitioning into skin tissue. The venous blood of the large intestine belongs to the portal vein system and is supplied to the liver. In the rectum, the portal veins are connected to the regular veins of our body. They tend to become inflamed or swollen, and they sometimes bleed if the liver and the enterohepatic circulation are overloaded (haemorrhoids).

The ring folds of a healthy large intestine alternately contract strongly, kneading the intestinal contents until a powerful forward movement (propulsion) announces the impulse to defecate and pushes the chymus down into the rectum. The discharge process forms autonomously and can only temporarily be stopped deliberately.

The Immune System of the Intestine

The tonsils are located at the entrance and back of the throat, and at the palate. They monitor infections in the nasopharyngeal cavity and fight them effectively. The defensive system of the appendix of the caecum similarly monitors the potentially unhealthy settlement of germs that would make us ill. The inner layer of the small intestine is characterized by tightly interspersed lymph cell nests, similar to a leopard's skin. In connection with the dense network of lymphatic vessels and lymph nodes, this layer forms the immune system of our intestine. Lymphocytes are produced in the bone marrow. To learn their skills for the immune system, they 'go to school' in the lymph cell nets of the intestinal mucosa. About 10 % of them pass the examinations for suitability for use in our immune system, followed by migration from the intestine into the lymph nodes, blood and tissues. A healthy milieu in the intestine and in our intestinal mucosa, and a balanced intestinal flora, are vital for competent immune defence not only in the intestine, but also in all mucous membranes throughout the body.

The Intestinal Flora

It includes the entirety of all microorganisms, bacteria, fungi and single-cell organisms (protozoa, amoebas, lamblia, etc.). The intestinal flora comprises an immense, complex ecosystem of bacteria that live in symbiotic community with the human body. The excreted bacteria mass makes up 30 % of the dry mass of stool. It has been determined that 10 to 100 trillion bacteria are living inside us, while our bodies comprise approx. 15 trillion cells. Most bacteria live without oxygen (anaerobic), some can use oxygen but do not have to, and others can only reproduce with oxygen (aerobic flora). The bacterial settlement of the intestine starts at birth and develops on the basis of nutrition. Adults house about 500 to 1000 different types[2] with a total mass of 1 to 2 kilograms. The flora of the small intestine is much less developed[3] and consists of bacteria that partially require oxygen (facultatively anaerobic bacteria), such as enterococci and lactobacteria.[4] The large intestine holds almost only bacteria that live without oxygen (anaerobes), such as bacteroids, bifidus bacteria, eubacteria, clostridia, fusobacteria, ruminococci and roseburia. The bacterium *Escherichia coli* exists in versions that are healthful for us and that flourish in acidic stool milieu, as well as in several pathogenic germs that threaten to become active in an alkaline, putrefaction-dominated intestinal milieu.

The intestinal flora meets important tasks in the intestine. A healthy bacteria complex fights undesired bacteria, protozoa, worms and fungi with great efficiency, thus preventing infections[5] (colonisation resistance). Intestinal bacteria contribute to our immune system.[6,7] They digest carbohydrates of the fibre of plant food that would otherwise be indigestible, using them to produce the short-chained fatty acids acetic acid, propionic acid and butyric acid. These are very important as nutrients for the intestinal mucosa cells and prevent their mutation into cancer.[8] Vegetable food will cause fermentation with the formation of acid and the gases hydrogen, methane and carbon dioxide. In mostly animal-based, protein-rich food, putrefaction processes will be dominant. In addition to the short-chained fatty acids, putrefaction will also lead to the formation of branched-chain fatty acids and an alkaline milieu under formation of thiols, amines, indoles, toxic hydrogen sulphide and nitrogen. The intestinal flora has an effect on body weight, since it has a great influence on the type of food resorption. The flora of overweight persons contains mostly bacteria of the Firmicutes type, while weight reduction will increase the share of bacteroids. Bacteria-free slim mice into whom the intestinal content of overweight mice was implanted would gain weight despite reduced food intake.[9,10,11]

Regulation of the Digestive System

We cannot deliberately control the nervous system – called the vegetative or autonomous nervous system – that regulates the digestive system. The nervous system is controlled by two antagonists: the sympathetic nervous system, which developed first (Chinese *Yang*) and is controlled by segments of the spinal cord; and the parasympathetic system (Chinese *Yin*), which controls its antagonist and keeps it within its borders. This is controlled by the centres of the brain stem via the nervus vagus. The sympathetic nervous system dominates with regard to activity, alertness, fighting and stress, while the parasympathetic system dominates at rest, sleep, digestion and recovery. Only when both systems are working in dynamic interaction can the digestive system work properly. Stress, overwork, sleeplessness or any other kind of disorderly lifestyle will block the digestive process, impairing peristalsis and production of the digestive juices. Flatulence, cramps, constipation or diarrhoea are possible symptoms. Domination of the parasympathetic system is rare today. The sympathetic nervous system contains many small brains (ganglia) that involuntarily control the autonomous functions. The most important are the coeliac ganglia, which consist of several nerve cell nodes placed in front of the spine in the upper abdomen. This 'abdominal brain' controls the functions of the upper abdominal organs down to the left large intestinal bend via the solar plexus (plexus solaris). The descending large intestine and the rectum are controlled by the bottom-most segments of the spinal cord and the nerve cell nodes (sympathicus ganglia) in the pelvis. This system is connected to the kidneys, urinary tract, prostate and sexual organs.

It's not surprising that this sensitive regulation is delicate and can be impaired by mental trauma or a lifestyle not in harmony with our biological nature.

Hormonal Regulation of Digestion

All hormones of the intestinal tract are formed in the mucosa.

Gastrin
The lower part of the stomach (antrum pylori) and the duodenum produce gastrin. Extension of the stomach wall or fragments of proteins in the stomach release gastrin, which stimulates the production of acidic gastric juice and the growth of the cells in the stomach wall until the acid content is above pH 3.

Cholecystokinin
When long-chained fatty acids, protein fragments and amino acids enter the small intestine, the cells of the small intestine's mucosa release the hormone cholecystokinin. This inhibits discharge of the stomach, triggers discharge of the gall bladder and stimulates growth and activity in the pancreas.

Secretin
When acidic stomach content enters the duodenum, the mucosa cells release the hormone secretin. This inhibits acid formation of the stomach, promotes activity in the pancreas and strongly stimulates production of bile in the liver.

GIP
When sugars (glucose), protein and fat fragments enter the small intestine, the cells of the mucosa produce the hormone GIP (glucose-dependant insulinotropic peptide). This hormone triggers insulin release of the islet cells of the pancreas and inhibits gastric-acid production.

Motilin
When the small intestine extends because it is newly filled, its nerve cells release the hormone motilin, which strongly stimulates peristalsis.

General messenger substances
Furthermore, the activity of the intestine is influenced by general messenger substances such as histamine, somatostatin and prostaglandin.

Diseases of the Oesophagus

Swallowing Problems

When swallowing, the tongue pushes a morsel of food into the throat. After this, the nasopharynx is sealed off by reflex, breathing is interrupted, the trachea is closed off and the oesophagus opened by the epiglottis. The peristaltic wave of the oesophagus is triggered, taking the morsel to the stomach. This complex process is controlled by the brain stem. Small strokes (transient ischaemic attacks, TIA) often impair this automatism, causing food to enter the lungs. In rare cases, this act of swallowing is impaired by bulges in the oesophagus (oesophageal hernia). The act of swallowing can only proceed in an orderly manner in a calm atmosphere during the meal and with enough time for careful chewing. Hasty eating and insufficient chewing will lead to inadequate preparation of the digestive tract. Starchy foods will not be digested sufficiently. This changes the intestinal flora and produces fermentation, bloatedness and the belching of gastric acid.

Reflux and Diaphragmatic Hernia

Overly frequent eating or snacking and nutrition with little vegetarian fresh food (raw food) can overextend the stomach until it sags into the abdominal cavity like a slack bag. The stomach entrance fold (cardia) slackens and extends until it slides up behind the sternum through the gap in the diaphragm (hiatus sliding hernia, diaphragmatic hernia). This causes bloatedness and belching of acidic gastric juice (reflux). The acid will burn the mucosa of the oesophagus, which is not equipped for this (reflux esophagitis).

Barrett Oesophagus (endobrachyoesophagus)

If nothing is done about the reflux, the mucosa of the oesophagus will partially convert to stomach mucosa, producing acid on its own, subject to frequently tormenting pain behind the sternum and in the upper abdomen. The oesophagus shortens because of this conversion. Persons with Barrett syndrome[12] suffer from an ulcer in the transformation zone. This affects approximately every 50th reflux patient. Two-thirds of the cases are men. [13,14] Chronic reflux is a cancer risk. Every 25th person affected will develop a preliminary stage of cancer (dysplasia), and every 100th Barrett patient will develop Barret cancer (adenocarcinoma).[15]

Therapy of Reflux and Barrett Syndrome

The production of gastric acid by the stomach mucosa is stimulated by the neurotransmitter histamine. This may be inhibited by certain medicines (ranitidine, H_2 blockers). Other medicines (Omeprazole) will block the enzyme sodium-potassium ATPase, virtually shutting down acid production. These medicines can produce dangerous side effects throughout the body, even in the brain, and should only be taken until the ulcer has healed. Sodium bicarbonate tablets buffer gastric acid for temporary relief

(Kaiser-Natron). Acid-absorbent gels can contain significant amounts of toxic aluminium and should be avoided. A good, natural remedy with temporary effect is potato juice: a small, raw potato, freshly passed through a centrifugal juicer together with two apples, sipped slowly. Very thin gruel also temporarily calms inflamed mucosa. Chamomile tea must be steeped very briefly and lightly. Peppermint tea also calms inflamed mucosa. Medicines may relieve symptoms and may be briefly required at the beginning of the therapy. However, they cannot heal reflux. The diet described in this book is designed to permanently heal the cause, and thus the reflux. Until the symptoms are gone, the strict, soothing dietary stages must be complied with, followed by several weeks of raw food diet. The stomach will slowly reduce its size and resume its healthy activity again. Barrett syndrome also heals if our diet is consistently followed for many months, even for one to two years. It is a path that is worth the effort.

Cancer of the Oesophagus (Oesophageal Carcinoma)

Oesophageal cancer mainly affects men older than 55 and is relatively rare. Eighty percent of carcinomas develop on the grounds of Barrett mucosa caused by reflux. Twenty percent of tumours grow higher up (squamous cell carcinoma), caused by regular ingestion of alcohol or hot drinks and smoking. Nutrition rich in animal products and coffee will additionally increase the risk. Symptoms of this cancer include a burning sensation when swallowing food, the sensation of a foreign body, permanent pain behind the sternum and tachycardia. By then, however, the tumour is usually already relatively large. When discovered early, it can be removed by endoscopic surgery (gastroscopy). Unfortunately, the tumour is often discovered late. This usually leads to chemotherapy and radiation therapy, followed by open removal of the oesophagus, a difficult piece of surgery that can only be performed in highly specialised centres. In an emergency, a spreading screen tube (stent) will be inserted to reduce problems with swallowing.

The prevention of oesophageal cancer is worthwhile[16,17,18,19,20,21] and can be achieved by rapid, permanent dietetic healing of reflux and conversion of nutrition to our vegetable fresh food: a high proportion (two-thirds) of raw food, fresh fruit at the beginning of every meal, nicotine abstinence, healthful drinks instead of alcohol and coffee, no overly hot food and drink, gentle steaming instead of roasting and frying, and reduction of cheese, eggs and dairy products to very small amounts. Plenty of sleep before midnight and lots of exercise every day are also important.[22,23,24,25,26]

Diseases of the Stomach

Gastritis

The inflammation may develop gradually from long-term harmful influences of a physical and mental nature, or acutely because of poisoning or infection.
Acute gastritis can be remedied quickly by taking the necessary care and resting, while chronic gastritis requires a patient and persistent effort to heal the damage to the digestive tissue.

The Over-Acidic Stomach (Chronic Gastritis)

Recurring stimulation from food or drink that is excessively hot or cold, strongly spiced, unnatural or irritating; from a lack of fresh nutrients; and from permanent nervous tension (stress), anger and discontent – particularly if these occur while eating – first causes the stomach to become overly acidic, with inflamed mucosa, unnaturally stimulated hunger, acidic belching, a cramping feeling after eating, and a burning, sore feeling when the stomach is empty.
Frequent, hasty, excessive meals and food rich in irritants, possibly combined with nicotine, alcohol, coffee and confectionery, will make the condition worse. If the condition continues for long, potentially dangerous ulcers may occur in the stomach, the oesophagus or the duodenum. Medicines that reduce gastric acid can reduce the symptoms at first. However, they will not heal the cause of the chronic gastritis. If they are taken for an extended period, they may have very dangerous adverse effects. They should be taken for short periods only (i.e. until the ulcer has healed).

The Acid-Deficient, Slack Stomach

If the irritation as described continues for a very long time, the stomach may become exhausted and turn into a low-acidic, slack stomach that will drop into the abdominal cavity like a sack, emptying slowly and with difficulty. Its content will start to disintegrate because of its long retention. Mild belching, a feeling of pressure and bloatedness, and flatulence up to severe distension are the consequences.

The lack of disinfecting acid permits pathogenic bacteria to enter the stomach, duodenum, small intestine and bile ducts, leading to the development of inflammations in the duodenum, the liver, the gall bladder and the large intestine (wrong bacteria settlement). This common digestion impairment (digestion dyspepsia) with distension after every meal, constipation and diarrhoea crises is a sign of the presence of the wrong bacteria, where the body-compatible healthy bacteria have been increasingly overgrown and displaced by fermentation- or putrefaction-causing strains, and sometimes by fungi. This is the soil on which stomach cancer ultimately can easily develop.
Chronic colitis also usually starts in this kind of degenerated gastrointestinal milieu. Liver diseases (e.g. epidemic jaundice), the common weak liver due to obesity, regular alcohol consumption, and chronic gall problems often coincide with chronic, low-acid gastritis and a chroni-

cally inflamed intestine. Therefore the liver and its enzymes always must be examined in case of gastrointestinal problems, in order to exclude the possibility of liver damage.

Colonisation of the Stomach by *Helicobacter Pylori*

The best-known bacterium that plays a role in bacterial miscolonization of the stomach is *Helicobacter pylori*. This small, curved bacterium can move in the stomach mucosa with flagellas and will find protection in the diseased, acid-reduced mucosa. *Helicobacter pylori* produces a toxin that stimulates gastric-acid formation. Helicobacter thus maintains gastritis, increases it, and produces stomach and duodenal ulcers. In 80 % of the patients suffering from a gastric ulcer (ulcus gastrici) and 90 % of the patients suffering from a duodenal ulcer (ulcus duodeni), this bacterium flourishes in the stomach. Although there are also persons with Helicobacter who have no ulcers at all, nine out of ten persons with gastritis have this bacterium in their stomach mucosa. Helicobacter is said to cause stomach cancer. However, it has been scientifically proven that only every thousandth carrier of Helicobacter will develop a stomach carcinoma, which means that Helicobacter can only be one of multiple causes.[27,28,29]

Helicobacter can often be temporarily eliminated by antibiotic therapy in combination with gastric-acid-blocking medication (eradication). However, this does not heal the cause, and chronic gastritis and reflux will recur. The vitamin C content of the stomach mucosa is particularly high in healthy persons, and reduced if Helicobacter is present. The dietetic healing of chronic gastritis can be helped by taking 4 × 500 mg of vitamin C per day.

Stomach Cancer

Around the world, stomach carcinoma is the second most common tumour in humans. In Central Europe, this type of cancer has been receding since the 1930s, as compared to other carcinomas. This is explained by the widespread use of refrigerators and the increased consumption of fresh fruit and vegetables, instead of salted meat and preserves. In Germany, every fifth cancer is a stomach carcinoma,[30,31] which affects five of every hundred thousand persons per year (men in two-thirds of all cases, often around 50 years of age).

In addition to chronic gastritis with gastric ulcer and *Helicobacter pylori*, a high nitrite content of food is one of the most important causes. Nitrites are found in high concentrations in salted meat and sausages, and also in preserves, sprayed vegetables and lettuces, and low-quality drinking water. Nitrites turn into nitrates in the stomach, which are carcinogenic. Smoking also increases the risk of stomach cancer. In case of chronic gastritis, the mucosa can change until it resembles intestinal mucosa. Such locations are particularly at risk for cancer. Benign adenomas also have a cancer occurrence of 30 %.[29] In case of iron deficiency and colonisation by *Helicobacter pylori*, the risk of stomach cancer is increased.[32] About every thirtieth chronic gastric ulcer will become cancerous. There is a certain hereditary role in the occurrence of stomach cancer. Other congenital factors play a role as well. People with blood type A have a slightly higher stomach cancer risk.[33] A clear increase of fruit and vegetables in the food will lower cancer risk significantly.[17,20] The higher the vitamin C level in the blood, the lower the stomach cancer risk.[34] Overweight persons with a lack of exercise will develop stomach cancer more frequently. Enjoying fruit several times per day, vegetables and a strong reduction of animal-based food protects against stomach cancer, as does abstinence from smoking, coffee[35,36] and alcohol.[21,22,23,24,25] Coffee produces chronic gastritis. Roasted substances, as well as the strongly oxidising contents of methyl xanthine, methylthioxal and hydrogen superoxide, potentiate each other in the production of free radicals and increase cancer risk in general.

The following foods are especially protective: all fruits and vegetables, garlic, raw onions, fresh lemons, broccoli, kale, fresh tomatoes, whole wheat, whole barley, linseed, all enjoyed raw if possible. All other fruits and vegetables will also decisively protect from cancer.[37,38] Careful cooking will reduce this protective effect by about 50 %.[39]

It is tragic that stomach cancer does not produce any symptoms while in its early stages. Only much later will patients complain of feeling bloated, and even later of persistent pain, lack of appetite and nausea. Therefore stomach cancer is usually discovered only during preventive gastroscopy or as a result of inflammation and ulcers. Anaemia and thrombosis in superficial veins may accompany stomach cancer.[40]

If a stomach carcinoma is recognised early enough, when it is still limited to the mucosa, it can be removed during a gastroscopy. Afterwards, we recommend long-term dietetic therapy to heal the cause in addition to oncology follow-up care.

Today if stomach cancer is recognised late, chemotherapy is recommended, followed by removal of the stomach and a bridge by means of a loop of the small intestine. These are severe, tragic operations. Preventing them is worth the effort.

Diseases of the Pancreas

Acute Pancreatitis

This is caused by gall stones that impair discharge. Acute pancreatitis produces severe pain in the upper abdomen, radiating into the back and causing nausea, vomiting, fever and constipation. Acute pancreatitis will usually heal with reduced food intake and infusions in a hospital.[41]
The blood-sugar level must be carefully monitored during the healing phase. A carefully designed diet that addresses the gallstone problem can be helpful.

Chronic Pancreatitis

Alcohol is the cause of chronic pancreatitis. Medical science notes that regular consumption of 16 g of pure alcohol per day is dangerous to the pancreas. This corresponds to 4 dl of beer, 1.1 dl of red wine, 4.5 dl of cider or 50 ml of brandy or spirits. A digestive drunk regularly will cause precipitation (sludge) to form in the fine pancreatic ducts. They produce chronic inflammation of the pancreas. Alcohol also damages the glandular cells directly and impairs the function of the sphincter of the excretory duct of the pancreas, causing the digestive enzymes activated in the small intestine to flow back and cause self-digestion of the pancreas. Every year in Germany 8,000 persons, 70 % of them men, are hospitalised as a result of chronic pancreatitis. Other causes are rare.

**Pancreatic Cancer
(Pancreatic Carcinoma)**

Every year, one of every 10,000 people develops pancreatic cancer. Scientifically recognised causes are alcohol, tobacco, nutrition rich in animal-based, salted or roasted food, and obesity. Daily consumption of more than two cups of coffee also significantly increases the risk of pancreatic cancer.[42] There are also indications for the same regarding daily intake of black tea. Usually the tumour is recognised too late to be removed. Cancer does not happen by accident. Diseases of the pancreas can be prevented.[33,34,35,36] Prevention is vital and can be achieved by protecting the pancreas and promoting the organism's ability to destroy the developing cancer by means of vegetarian nutrition with a raw food proportion of at least 70 %, and by abstinence from irritants such as alcohol, nicotine, coffee, sugar and salted, strongly roasted or grilled foods. Such abstinence will pay off.[43]

**Failure of the Pancreas
(Pancreas Insufficiency)**

Chronic inflammation or the congenital disease cystic fibrosis will prevent the pancreas from producing enzymes at sufficient amounts, so that the intestine is unable to properly digest food (malabsorption). The stool contains fat, and it floats. Light fresh vegetarian food reduces the enzyme demand considerably and improves the symptoms. Enzyme preparations are also available. Endocrine pancreatic insufficiency causes diabetes.

Diseases of the Intestine

Duodenal Ulcer (Ulcus duodeni)

Chronic gastritis with bacterial miscolonization of the stomach as described in the section on stomach diseases is the most significant cause of duodenal ulcers. Its symptoms include hypersensitivity to food irritating the stomach, and severe pain in the middle of the upper abdomen (epigastrium). There is often severe pain below the liver, on the right, radiating to the right into the back, causing loss of appetite and weight loss. A duodenal ulcer may break open again recurrently after initially scarring over, though it will rarely become cancerous. If the condition persists, the duodenum deforms and tightens. Permanent healing is possible only through dietetic healing of the chronic gastritis.

Intestinal Catarrh (Enteritis, Colitis, Fermentation, Rot)

Constipation and diarrhoea are the most common intestinal problems that reflect an inadequate intestinal function, in terms of both intestinal peristalsis and the bacterial milieu. The patient suffering from intestinal disease feels heavy, bloated and distended. Discharge is difficult and alternates with stomach aches and days of diarrhoea attacks and strong gas formation. Such diarrhoea may occur after eating specific foods, after excitement or fatigue, and in anticipation of deadlines, exams or other events. Diarrhoea may also occur without any evident reason at all, at an apparently consistent alternation with constipation. These are the usual symptoms of catarrh of the large intestine with bacterial miscolonization

General well-being suffers under such conditions. Moods swing and the patient is irritated, often depressed. The patient feels tired, tends to be sensitive to the weather, and has headaches and migraines. Circulation in the hands and feet is poor. A large number of patients suffering from rheumatism also have problems with their large intestine (see Manual no. 10, for patients with rheumatism and arthritis). It should now be evident how much of a strain the large intestine can place on the overall health as an interference focus and source of toxins. If the healthy intestinal bacteria are missing, utilisation of food, removal of toxins and detoxification are impaired. There are not enough protective substances, ferments and vitamin groups (e.g. vitamins B_{12}, B_2, K), which are necessary for proper conversion of food to body substance and energy. This leads to putrefaction or fermentation, especially when overeating. The food remains in the intestine for too long and disintegrates. The toxins pass through the irritated and weakened intestinal walls and enter the blood stream, causing allergic defence reactions and damaging all body tissues.

The main cause of this kind of impaired intestinal function lies in poor nutrition, now widespread. An impaired intestinal function is an expression of general tissue weakening from lack of vital protective and vital substances, trace elements and enzymes that are only present in sufficient amounts and at the right ratio to each other in a harmonious, natural diet. The immense network of capillaries, the pervasive tender connective tissue (matrix) with its basic substance, is embedded in a molecular network of proteoglycans which controls the exchange of information and substance among all cells of the organism. The finely-built, coordinated digestive cells first suffer from nutritional damage. If an acute, general disease is added to this (e.g. an infection such as jaundice, gastric flu or travelling dysentery, cold or mental trauma), acute or chronic colitis develops. The most frequently prescribed medicines for diarrhoea or constipation only make the situation worse, as does the generally prescribed semi-solid food and the bland diet that deplete the organism of important substances and that never improve intestinal flora. Climate cures and fastidious avoidance of any effort do not help either. Colitis can be permanently healed, but only by returning to a healthy lifestyle and nutrition. The diet must be carefully adjusted both mechanically and in substance to the condition of the digestive system. The will to be healed must also be present.

Severe forms of colitis with ulcers of the mucous membranes, and massive, bloody and slimy stool (infectious colitis, colitis ulcerosa or Crohn's disease), often require hospitalisation and daily monitoring by a doctor. Therapy can continue on an outpatient basis after such crises. Careful support and thorough consultation by a doctor that enables the patient to correctly perform dietetic therapy are the most important prerequisites for healing.

Constipation and Diarrhoea

The lazy intestine requires fresh food in the form of fibre- and cellulose-rich raw vegetables (whole if possible), fruit and whole-grain foods. Consistent application of longer and repeated pure raw food periods will restore normal intestinal activity and digestion, and the intestine will recover its ability to employ the food supplied economically. The patient will then experience, and especially in advanced years, that the body can function normally with a much lower food supply than before, and simultaneously develop a great ability to function satisfactorily.

Diarrhoea requires protection of the irritated intestine as far as possible. The raw food parts are consumed as juice or puree. Further mitigation is offered by an addition of vegetable gruel or grain gel ('enveloping' the fresh juices).

Although diarrhoea and constipation are opposite problems, they often alternate in the same patients at regular intervals. Both are consequences of continuous nutritional errors and the pervasive impairment of the microbial milieu of the intestine, the metabolism and the detoxification process of the body. Infection and mental-conflict situations often trigger the problem. Constipation and diarrhoea are also both expressions of impaired bowel movement (slackness or cramping) and impaired intestinal milieus (bacterial inflammation, poisoning with toxins of pathogenic germs). As a consequence, the intestine – and also the immune system, the stomach, the liver, the pancreas and the pervasive soft connective tissue with its basic substance (matrix) – will suffer until the entire organism enters a phase of chronic slagging from toxins and rheumatism, arteriosclerosis, migraine, Alzheimer's disease, diabetes mellitus, kidney damage, etc. make their appearance. Both extremes, diarrhoea and constipation, require the same basic line of treatment for the following reasons: detoxing, purification, reorganizing lifestyle function and order, and above all pursuing a healing diet of the highest quality.

Of course, this basic diet must be carefully adjusted to the different forms of manifestation of the gastrointestinal disease, as reflected in the diet types I–V and the recipe part.

Laxatives
Swelling agents stimulate intestinal activity by increasing stool volume. Lactulose influences the intestinal flora by promoting the population of lactobacilli which, while not harmful, do not solve the problem. Senna-containing and chemical laxatives should be avoided, since they further paralyse and slacken the intestine. Longer and repeated fresh food periods, in contrast, will almost always lead to normal, consistent intestinal activity and digestion, to recovery of the full use of the foods by the intestine and regular, healthy stool. See 'Permanent Diet for Frequent Constipation', page 59.

It is very important to take meals calmly and in a relaxed atmosphere. Rest afterwards and hike for at least one hour per day. The movement and rhythm of walking will regulate the motility of the intestine and help prevent cancer.[19,22,23,24,25] The body compress improves and invigorates the intestinal function and promotes circulation.
Very often the intestine expresses unresolved mental conflicts in life, or unprocessed traumas that must be addressed in addition to dietetic therapy.

Intestinal Putrefaction and Fermentation, Bacterial Miscolonization

The intestinal flora is a dynamic bacterial ecosystem. The first bacteria that enter the intestine will flourish from birth. The first bacteria that colonise the intestine are enterobacteria, *Escherichia coli* and streptococci. Children born by caesarean section initially have an unnatural intestinal flora. The intestine of breast-fed children will mostly be settled by lactic-acid-producing bacteria in the first weeks: bifidobacteria and lactobacilli. These produce lactic acid, acidifying the milieu in the intestine. The stool becomes yellow and grainy. The lactic acid makes it difficult for pathogenic bacteria to enter and thereby protects from infections. In the intestine of bottle-fed children who receive processed, unnatural powdered milk, the intestinal flora is similar to that of an adult, with an alkaline milieu and dark stool. The intestine of a healthy adult contains about 100 trillion bacteria (about 500 types), mostly bacteria that can reproduce without oxygen (anaerobes). The most important types are bacteroides, firmicutes, proteobacteria and actinobacteria and, in very small amounts, bifidobacteria, eubacteria, clostridia, fusobacteria, ruminococci and rosaburia. In contrast, far fewer bacteria live in the small intestine, mainly those which can flourish with and without oxygen (facultative anaerobes), such as enterococci and lactobacilli. Healthy *Escherichia coli* strains flourish in an acidic stool milieu. Other coli types are pathogens, including enterohaemorrhagic, enteroinvasive and enterotoxic coli types. Pathogenic bacteria, fungi, amoebae, lamblias and worm parasites can only become pathogenic if the intestinal flora is strongly impaired, since a healthy flora will keep them from developing (colonisation resistance). Food that is rich in carbohydrates and fibre will promote the growth of fermenting bacteria, which form harmless carbon dioxide, hydrogen and methane gases as well as the odorous butyric acid that is very important for the nutrition of the intestinal mucosa cells and protects them from cancerous mutations.

In contrast, proteins are broken down by the obligate anaerobic flora, which may become dominant at a protein-rich diet. This will cause the production of toxic gases smelling of manure or rotting eggs, such as thiol, indole, hydrogen sulphide and small quantities of nitrogen gas.

Infections with such bacteria produce partially dangerous cases of colitis. The first of these is the bacterium *Clostridium difficile,* which is at home in hospitals and nursing homes (hospitalisation), since it has developed resistance to antibiotics and disinfectants, and causes a dangerous, pseudomembranose enterocolitis (a nosocomial infection).

Miscolonization of the Small Intestine

This causes partially massive digestive problems and food intolerances that lead to great suffering. The hydrogen breath test will show increased values. If this is the case, the diagnosis of miscolonization should be confirmed by a hydrogen breath test with lactose or fructose. Miscolonization of the small intestine often produces an intolerance of fructose (acquired fructose intolerance), since the fructose-utilising bacteria can reproduce quickly when ingesting fruit sugar (fruit, sweet vegetables), causing diarrhoea and nausea. If miscolonization of the small intestine is indicated, the weakened, irritated mucosa of the small intestine will also often overreact to histamine, which occurs in many foods. Initially, in these two situations, fructose or strongly histamine-containing foods must be avoided. If the miscolonization has pronounced carbohydrate-utilising bacteria types because large quantities of sugar- and starch-containing foods are being consumed, fungi- and particularly *Candida albicans* – will also begin to settle in the intestine. Uncontrolled growth of *Candida albicans* in the intestine is also common in infants fed on formula milk. In adults, growth of this yeast fungus may become so bad even without immune deficiency (AIDS) that the *Candida albicans* enters the blood stream and various organs (candidosis).

Intestinal Putrefaction

This results from a diet that is too rich in protein. The proteins consumed in excess are broken down by anaerobic intestinal bacteria, which then grow to an excessive extent because of poor nutrition. The intestinal mucosa's cells are fed insufficiently, since there is not enough fibre in the intestine and not enough fermenting bacteria to produce the short-chained fatty acids to feed them. The putrefaction gases are toxic to the mucosa and the metabolism, and they produce meteorism. The cancer risk is increased. Intestinal putrefaction is the most common cause of irritable bowel syndrome. The food is digested incompletely (lienteria), the stool becomes inert or falls apart and is discharged explosively when the rectum is inflamed (proctitis). The discharges smell rotten, are acidic and cause soreness. The veins of the rectum also often become inflamed in this situation (haemorrhoids).

Therapy of Bacterial Miscolonization

To treat intestinal putrefaction, the protein content in the patient's diet must be strongly reduced (i.e. starting with the raw apple diet and continuing with the raw food diet). Fermentation processes, however, use high-quality proteins, starting with the sour milk diet if the patient is not intolerant of milk, followed by the raw food diet with green leaves, raw vegetables and lettuces, and fresh soy, sour milk, buttermilk, quark and low-fat soft cheese. Raw vegetables that do not cause flatulence should be chosen. They are best enjoyed passed through a centrifugal juicer as fresh juices first (diet II A – C). Grain is used only if finely mixed as wholemeal, gel or gruel, as well as crisp bread, wholemeal rusk and sprout bread. Acidic, low-sugar fruits should be chosen, such as berries, and specifically blueberries that contain the flavonoid group of anthrocyanes which counter inflammation, modulate the immune system and fight pathogenic germs. Sugar and white flour are prohibited.

To monitor the process of healing of intestinal diseases, the bacterial culture and a precise review of the intestinal flora have turned out to be helpful. Apart from the type and distribution of the physiological intestinal flora, one should look for pathological germs (cocci, Welch-Fraenkel, proteus), parasites, amoeba types, lamblia, etc. and also determine the degree of fermentation or rot (pH and organic acids, etc.). By the administration of normal, living coli germs via the mouth and intestine, the intestinal milieu can often be adjusted more quickly (symbiosis control), and effective substances can be better formed by increased growth of physiological coli strains. To further improve the intestinal condition, additional vitamin intake (vitamins A, B, and C) has proven valuable, as has the use of healing earths and vegetable carbon. To disinfect the intestine, you can also use the natural antibiotic effect of garden cress and nasturtium salad (3 times daily 20–30 g). Treatment for parasites and infection should be performed by a doctor.

Natural yoghurt, served with wholemeal, potatoes, fresh fruit (or fruit juices) and other foods is the ideal combination. With its intestine-stimulating effect, it has a positive effect on both constipation and diarrhoea and is also both nourishing and thirst-quenching. Milk-souring products belong with whole food if tolerated. They have a dietetic task as well. Yoghurt is preferably produced from gently cooked and self-pasteurised, certified raw milk. Pure yoghurt bacteria cultures are not possible without prior heating, while the sour milk of raw milk produced in hot weather – if of impeccable quality – retains most qualities of raw milk. Yoghurt, sour and buttermilk contain certain lactic-acid bacteria typical for the types named, and in moderate amounts have a healing effect on the bacterial milieu of the intestine, promote digestion, prevent flatulence and permit milk supply in soured form to all those many gastrointestinal patients who react allergically (flatulence, cramps, etc.) to sweet milk. Doctors in tropical countries know about the healing effect of sour milk on the tender digestive system of infants during the weaning period, and the healing effect of a few days of buttermilk diet in acute intestinal infections. In Germany, health-food stores offer special sour-milk products that are preferable to ordinary yoghurt (e.g. Bioghurt, Lünebest-Spezial Joghurt and Sanoghurt). All sour-milk types may be enjoyed in moderation. During the dietary phase, the doctor will monitor the quantity and duration of consumption.

Appendicitis

Inflammation of the appendix of the caecum is almost always the consequence of a permanent irritation of the large intestine, putrefaction and constipation, and is caused by unhealthy food.

At the first sign of *acute* pain in the lower right abdomen, sometimes coinciding with fever, a doctor should be called immediately. This is an emergency situation. Laxatives are strictly forbidden. Do not drink anything and lie still until a doctor comes and determines if surgery is required.

Chronic appendicitis can usually be healed by neural therapy. Only in the rare cases where this is not possible will surgery be necessary to permit final healing and to prevent the spread throughout the body of infectious substances from the inflammation. The pain attacks that occur at more or less regular intervals with chronic appendicitis will often recede if a healing diet (full fasting or fresh juice diet) is begun immediately. The attacks will become rarer and less severe and will heal slowly and without surgery. A doctor must be consulted every time there is a pain attack. Afterwards cold Priessnitz compresses on the stomach will help calm the process.

Meteorism

This is not an illness, but a very irritating and often painful side effect of chronic gastrointestinal disease. It may occur when there is an excess of acidity, but even more when there is an acid-deficient atropic stomach, liver or pancreas disease, enteritis or (especially) chronic colitis. Flatulence merely means gas collection in the stomach, small or large intestine. This is rarely caused by swallowing air (aerophagia), a nervous habit, produced by suppressed feelings, 'swallowed anger', overly hot food in an irritable stomach. The vast majority of people suffering from flatulence suffer from a pervasive change in the intestinal bacterial flora (miscolonization). Years of poor nutrition, irritating food, regular ingestion of hot spices, excessive amounts of table salt, coffee, roasted products, sweets, and especially alcohol and nicotine form the basis of this degeneration of the digestive system. Insufficient movement and circulation in the abdominal organs only make matters worse. Jaundice or acute intestinal infection, particularly treatment with antibiotic medication, and sulfonamides or other disinfectants may greatly alter the intestinal bacteria and promote miscolonization and dysbiosis. The consequence of this, as described above, is deficient production of digestive juices and a vitamin deficiency due to insufficient utilisation of the food. If the stomach mucosa has atrophied, the intrinsic factor for the resorption of vitamin B_{12} is missing in the last section of the small intestine (ileum), just as for the vitamin B_{12} that is produced by the bacteria in the large intestine, leading to the menace of anaemia and neurological damage. All of these problems will often cause only 'bloatedness' in the patient, flatulence that either starts after eating or that persists all day and into the night, tormenting him or her and possibly turning into severe pain attacks with irritation of the peritoneum.

Often certain foods will suddenly cause flatulence. Some of them are hydrogenated fats, refined oils, chocolate, sweet whole milk, cabbage (much more flatulence- inducing when cooked than raw), fresh bread, individual fruit types, confectionery, fatty meat, cheese and hard-boiled eggs. These are individually various sensitivities expressing partial damage to the digestive secretion or excess of specific, abnormal, pathogenic bacterial strains in the intestine, and usually not an allergic phenomenon. These produce acute gas in a special nutritional milieu, depending on food and bacteria type: odourless in the case of fermentation, and smelling very much like sulphur in case of putrefaction. A constipated intestine with contents that are putrefying or fermenting is a treasure trove of pathogenic bacteria and a source of flatulence and chronic poisoning of the blood.

Treatment directives for meteorism

Meteorism is overcome by removing the basic disease, as described in the individual disease groups. Regeneration of the pathogenic intestinal bacteria is made possible by whole food nutrients and in particular by supplying the protective substances and ferments that only natural food can ensure. *Degraded food means degraded intestinal flora!* No disinfection, no antibiotic therapy can heal in the long term when the daily food does not provide the proper terrain.

First, the intestine should be emptied with a chamomile enema or an intestinal bath (hydrocolon therapy). This is followed by a day of complete rest for the intestine with ingestion of only flatulence-reducing teas, followed by a transition to the juice diet and then, depending on the duration of the diet (varying from individual to individual), to the mash diet. Preference should be given to buttermilk, whey, yoghurt, flaxseed, barley and rice gruel, or to whole-wheat gel, carrot, beetroot, cabbage juice and raw potato juice taken several times a day in small sips. Other possibilities are sauerkraut juice and sea water and, among the fruit juices, the sour types mixed with gruel (sweet juices of grapes, sweet plums, peach, etc. will cause fermentation flatulence because of their sugar content). Intestinal cleaning with chamomile enemas should take place every 1–2 days during the juice diet. The importance of adequate salivation and chewing must be explained to the patient. Body compresses, deep-tissue massage and breathing exercise are valuable supports.

If flatulence is accompanied by diarrhoea, an apple day should follow the tea day (see Diet II A), and possibly a buttermilk day, particularly in the hot season or in a tropical climate. Healing earth *between* meals, with anti-flatulence tea, binds gas and soothes, especially before sleeping at night. Drinking a large quantity of liquid with meals is not beneficial. Raw green-leaved vegetables are especially valuable but must, in our experience, be given in the form of juice or fine mash for a longer time than other raw vegetables. If possible, compost fertilised green leafy vegetables are preferable. All *cabbage types* are tolerated without flatulence in the raw juice form. Whether the cabbage is cooked or not mashed, the digestive system would respond by forming gas as a result of the cellulose content, and digest it slowly. Whole grain is well tolerated when taken consistently and chewed carefully, first as gruel and whole wheat gel, later as sprouted wheat, and then followed by wheat meal and wholemeal bread. Whole grain must replace wheat flour, and honey in moderation replaces sugar. Sweet whole milk can be drunk only in small amounts after the first strict conversion diet, while sour milk, yoghurt, whey and buttermilk are permitted earlier. Teas are best drunk with lemon or a little cream instead of milk.

Rest and relaxation before and after eating are very important. Life conflicts and stress at work are often the main promoters of meteorism and prevent normalisation of the digestion. They must be observed and resolved. A tendency to feel cold must be overcome by movement and suitable water applications, dry brushing, etc.

Summary: Meteorism is a consequence of pathogenic changes to the intestinal bacteria. It can only be overcome by a maximum supply of fresh nutrients in food and by healing chronic constipation. Rest and thorough emptying of the intestine should precede treatment with the healing diet. Degraded, irritating food must be avoided in the future, the intestinal flora continually regenerated and the circulation invigorated by daily walking, swimming and cold water applications.

Irritable Bowel Syndrome

This term summarises a group of functional intestinal problems that are harmless but imitate the symptoms of various intestinal diseases. Irritable bowel syndrome (IBS) is very common. In Western industrial countries, 15 % of the population suffers from IBS, as does every second patient who sees a gastrointestinal specialist.

Irritable bowel syndrome is also called irritable colon.

The patient suffers from pain or discomfort in the abdominal area. Stool habits change, for which a structural or biochemical cause has been excluded. The intestine of these persons is generally very sensitive and tends to develop flatulence, diarrhoea or constipation; or to suffer from both, in addition to abdominal cramps (spastic colon).
Some of these people also suffer from chronic pain in the pelvis or the muscles, fascia and tendons (fibromyalgia) and are mentally and emotionally exhausted. The symptoms often grow worse after ingestion of dairy products or wheat bread, although milk protein allergy, actual lactose intolerance or gluten sensitivity could not be documented.
It is scientifically recognised that bacterial miscolonization is present to a degree in irritable bowel syndrome. The US association of gastroenterologists has issued the Rom-II-Konsus diagnosis criteria for the diagnosis of irritable bowel syndrome, which affects the frequency and type of the symptoms and the influence of food intake and stool discharge. Diagnosis of irritable bowel syndrome is only permitted if the following do not reveal any pathological results: ultrasound examination of the abdomen; gastroscopy and colonoscopy; a profile of lab examinations; a deep biopsy of the small intestine to exclude coeliac disease; hydrogen breath tests to exclude lactose or fructose intolerance and severe miscolonization of the small intestine; and a test for sorbit intolerance.

The cause of irritable bowel syndrome is much discussed at congresses. Slight gluten sensitivity is recognised as a partial cause if this has been confirmed by testing with a gluten-free diet.[43]
Every fourth patient developed irritable bowels after colitis or antibiotic therapy.
It is also suspected that food aromas to which the enterochromaffine cells of the intestine react promote irritable bowel syndrome.

It is recognised today that irritable bowel syndrome comes with a slight miscolonization of the small intestine. Peristalsis and transport of the food bolus is slowed. Insufficiently digested parts of the food enter the lower part of the small intestine, serving as nourishment for bacteria having migrated from the large intestine. Fermentation or putrefaction gases irritate the small and large intestine, causing the irritation.[44]

Medicine treats this problem by reducing the short-chained carbohydrates and alcohols in the diet. Furthermore, peppermint oil capsules, fibre preparations and cramp-relieving medicines are prescribed, as well as water soluble fibres such as flea seeds (psyllium seeds) or calming balm leaf extracts. Short term antibiotic therapies, after which the symptoms will recur immediately, are also administered. In IBS, the homoeopathic remedy colocynthis in the two hundredth potency immediately and reliably removes cramps in children and adults who had been writhing with pain before.

Our experience has shown that irritable bowel syndrome can be reliably healed. The therapy of the cause (i.e. bacterial miscolonization) corresponds to that of meteorism, as described above.

Coeliac Disease (Herter's Disease)

In 1909, the German physician Herter described a disease that he called 'intestinal infantilism', since the children studied were badly retarded in their development. The children suffered from chronic diarrhoea with malabsorption (lack of absorption of nutrients in the intestine), causing anaemia and many dangerous deficiency symptoms. The intestinal mucosa of these children was atrophied, so that the mucous membrane's villi were degenerated and could no longer utilise the food. In the beginning, the problem in these children was believed to be caused by the congenital lack of an enzyme needed to absorb gluten. Gluten is a part of the glue protein gliadin that occurs in wheat, spelt and rye, and in small amounts in oats and green spelt grain.

Through of much lesser severity, gluten intolerance is now present in many adults and is called *gluten-sensitive enteropathy,* Herter-Heubner's disease, or *domestic* or *non-tropical sprue*. Today we know that it is over-sensitivity to gluten. Gluten causes an inflammation of the intestinal mucosa that leads to atrophy and malabsorption. The adult will also suffer from weight loss, fatty diarrhoea, vomiting, lack of appetite, extreme fatigue and melancholy. Diabetes mellitus type I is 5–10 % more common in patients with coeliac disease. They also develop non-Hodgkin lymphoma (lymph node cancer) more frequently and, it is suspected, carcinomas of the intestinal tract, especially lymph node cancer (lymphoma) of the small intestine.

The components of the glue protein to which the immune system of the intestine reacts allergically depend on the cereal type. Wheat must be differentiated into α, β and ω gliadin-C-C allergen. Barley has hordenin and amylase inhibitors IAM1 and CMb. Oats, which only rarely cause allergic reactions, contain the avenines A, E and F. Rye contains secalin. Wheat and barley allergens also cause bakers' asthma. Gluten-free cereal types include corn, rice and millet. However, these are contaminated with gluten in some mills. According to EU regulations, they must be marked 'may contain traces of gluten'. Products guaranteed to be gluten-free are available from the trade for those suffering from coeliac disease. In the EU, they are marked with a special logo (e.g. a barred grain).

Gluten sensitivity in adults has become much more common today. It depends on nutrition and the quality of the grain supply. In Denmark, every thousandth person suffers from gluten-induced symptoms, while in the USA the symptoms affect every three-hundredth person. It has been calculated that about every three-thousandth person worldwide suffers from gluten-induced symptoms. However, every hundredth American and every five-hundredth German will react to gluten allergy tests.[46] It is assumed that the risk of developing coeliac disease is higher if cereals are fed early in infancy. Adults usually develop it in the fourth decade of their lives. The condition is more common in women than in men. The cause of gluten sensitivity has been explained more satisfactorily in recent years. The affected persons suffer from an impairment of the intestinal mucosa barrier. Gluten proteins may pass through the mucosa into the intestinal muscle layer (endomysium). There the enzyme transglutaminase converts gliadin into peptides, which trigger a local immune reaction and activate T-cells of the enteral immune system. The T-cells attack the intestinal mucosa. It has also been documented that miscolonization of the intestine – especially when the yeast fungus *Candida albicans* has settled in the intestine or impairment of the intestinal flora has occurred because of infection, alcohol consumption or stress factors – will increase the activity of transglutaminase and thus promote development of coeliac disease.[47] It is not certain yet whether there is also a congenital cause of coeliac disease. A number of histocompatibility antigens are definitely found in the case of coeliac disease. However, they also occur in 98 % of the healthy population.[48] Gliadin contains a particularly large amount of the amino acids proline and glutamine in its peptide chains. They cause the mucosa cells of the intestine to produce increased amounts of the histocompatibility antigens of the HLA-classes I, DR and DQ on their surfaces. Since the peptides of gliadin contain a particularly high amount of glutamine, the enzyme transglutaminase leads to the production of particularly large amounts of glutamine acid, which binds to the HLA-DQ-antigen of the cell surface and activates the CD4$^+$ helper cells of the enteral immune system. These helper cells activate the inflammatory substances interferon γ, tumour necrosis factor α and the interleukins 1 and 6. B-cells of the immune system produce different antibodies to counter gliadin. Auto-antibodies against endogenic structures and against the enzyme tissue transglutaminase are also found in this disease. Therefore, coeliac disease is considered a mixture of allergy and autoimmune disease. However, the scope of the autoimmune component (i.e. the reaction of the immune system against the endogenic structures) is essential for the severity of the disease, which will ultimately cause destruction of the intestinal mucosa cells (apoptosis). This leads to a loss of mucosa villi and insufficient resorption of food.

The appearance of gliadin antibodies does not prove coeliac disease at this stage. The exclusion of the histocompatibility antigens involved excludes it through a very elaborate process. The proof of antibodies against tissue transglutaminase is a strong indicator of coeliac disease, but the diagnosis can only be confirmed by means of a biopsy of the small intestine's mucosa. Since more and more cases of slight coeliac disease are occurring, new diagnosis guidelines[49] differentiate among three categories: symptomatic, subclinical and refractory coeliac disease. The mild symptoms are called an iceberg phenomenon, since such symptoms do not lead directly to the diagnosis. These patients suffer from stomach ache, sometimes even constipation, reduced calcium content in the bones (osteopenia), iron-deficiency anaemia and, in children, delayed growth and delayed puberty. The strong, actual sprue in adults was first observed in tropical climates: the Herter's disease of the adult. Some indications suggest that the cause of coeliac disease is a miscolonization of the intestine that is rooted in the widespread poor nutrition of children and adults.

Treatment of coeliac disease

It is important to treat anaemia first, immediately followed by a gluten-free, carefully composed plant-based diet rich in fresh food. The patients require a long, very careful treatment. Since 1927, when Dr. Bircher-Benner employed a raw diet to heal his first case of Herter's disease in a child, further research has produced further important information for patients with coelic disease. Supply of vitamin E, folic acid and other vitamins of the B-group encourage healing and increases the vitamin A and E content of the blood. The use of green leaves and vegetables is very important, as is the supply of unsaturated fatty acids in sunflower seeds, pure wheat sprout oil, flax eed oil, apples, bananas, strawberries and blueberries. *Wheat, rye, barley and oats in all forms are to be strictly avoided because of their gluten content. Spelt wheat contains a particularly high amount of gluten and must be strictly avoided as well.* Other grains (e.g. corn, millet, rice) must be of an origin that is guaranteed not to have been contaminated with gluten. They are well tolerated and important because of their vitamin B content. *Butter and animal based fats of all kinds* must be reduced. Since food utilisation is strongly reduced as a result of the pathogenically reduced digestive ability of the mucosa, all vital elements must be administered in a carefully maintained harmony and rich in vital substances. Only superior quality foods should be chosen. Degraded and unbalanced food must be avoided. A supply of protein in an easily absorbable form must be ensured. Concurrent intolerance of milk protein must be excluded, in which case lean milk, whey, buttermilk, and possibly protein milk (Ursa, Pelargon, etc.) are suitable. Lean quark (and other non-fat soft cheese types), soy, almond puree, sesame puree, green leaves and ripe bananas rich in vitamin E serve the same purpose. Sugars must come only from natural sources: fresh food, vegetables, and freshly broken-down, well-chewed cereal grains of permitted types. Patients with coeliac disease must comply with a carefully increasing raw food diet under observation of these directives, as described in Diet II A and III. Additionally, there must be temporary vitamin and mineral additions (calcium, phosphorus, iron, magnesium, zinc, selenium), depending on blood-analysis results. Sun lamps, body compresses, mild light arcs, water baths and careful handling of the often severely stressed psychological situation of the patients are all very important. *Every patient with coeliac disease must be treated by a doctor.*

Lactose Intolerance

Lactose (milk sugar) is contained in breast milk and milk of animal origin. It is made up of two sugar molecules (disaccharide), glucose and galactose, which must be split by the enzyme lactase in the small intestine to become re-absorbable. Lactose intolerance is not an allergy. New-born children have high lactase activity in the small intestine at birth in order to digest breast milk. The activity of this enzyme slowly declines afterwards. About three-fourths of all adults in the world are lactose intolerant. In all areas where dairy production has been in operation for a long time, the lactase activity in adults is more or less retained. This includes all of North America, central Europe, eastern Europe, northern Asia, Australia and New Zealand.

However, the residual activity of lactase is not the same in every person in these regions. If the quantity of sweet milk and sweet-milk products exceeds an individual threshold, undigested lactose will enter the large intestine. There it will be fermented into lactic acid by bacteria. The fermentation products are the gases methane and hydrogen, which cause unpleasant flatulence. The lactic acid osmotically draws water back into the intestine, causing diarrhoea. These symptoms are not always pronounced. If they are weak, degradation products and toxins from miscolonization by bacteria will produce various symptoms, such as a feeling of pressure, abdominal cramps, melancholy, aching limbs, inner unrest, vertigo, sweating, headache, fatigue, nervousness, sleeping problems, lack of concentration, and acne. These patients often suffer from a deficiency of vitamins, minerals and trace elements. They also suffer more frequently from infections. These atypical cases are referred to as lactose mal-digestion. In Germany, it is estimated that 10–25 % of the population suffers from lactose intolerance. If the problem is not recognised and persists, there can be damage to the small intestine's mucosa, as in coeliac disease, with partial degeneration of the villi. For people from Africa, South and Central America, Mexico, Japan, south Asia and other areas with few dairy products, lactose intolerance is not an illness; it is considered normal. Lactose intolerance[50] produces symptoms similar to those of fructose intolerance and irritable bowel syndrome.

The diagnosis is performed by a lactose-free diet lasting several days, followed by lactose exposure. If the result is not clear enough, a hydrogen breath test under lactose exposure may provide evidence of increased exhalation of hydrogen, which results from lactic acid fermentation. This would confirm the diagnosis. Further information may be blood sugar measurement during and after lactose exposure (blood sugar test), since the lack of degradation of lactose to glucose and galactose will cause the blood sugar to rise insufficiently. In persons with a strong lactase deficiency, the LCT-genotype[51] can be determined from buccal mucosa.

Treatment consists of strong reduction of lactose-containing foods. In addition to plant milks (rice, soy, almond, sesame), lactose-reduced dairy products are available commercially. Fermented dairy products such as sour milk and buttermilk contain very little lactose and already contain the enzyme lactase, so they are well tolerated. However, dairy products are not required for healthful nutrition.

Industrial products add lactose as a flavour enhancer. This applies to sausages and marinated meat, spice mixes, soup packs, cereal bars and breads, microwavable meals, pastry products, candy, ice cream, instant products and chocolate. Since 2005, foods containing lactose must be labelled. Small amounts as found in medicines or homoeopathic preparations are easily tolerated, since intolerance is not an allergy but rather depends on the dosage.
Lactose intolerance after intestinal infections can be healed by the proper diet.[52] Healing of the bacterial miscolonization will also improve lactose intolerance.

Fructose Intolerance

Intolerance of fruit sugar has become increasingly common in recent decades, since the food industry began adding fruit sugar to many preparations as a flavour enhancer and sweetening agent. Central European food currently contains 11–54 g of fruit sugar per person and day.[53] Congenital fructose intolerance with a genetic lack of enzyme is rare. Such children and adults will never be able to tolerate even small amounts of fruit sugar. Acquired fruit sugar intolerance has become common today. Scientific studies in various countries show that about one-third of all persons taking in 25 g or more of fructose per day will develop fructose malabsorption.[54,55,56] The share of persons with fructose malabsorption in the general population is about as high as that of patients with functional intestinal problems. This permits the conclusion that fructose malabsorption is a 'normal' accompanying problem of functional intestinal problems due to widespread poor nutrition and bacterial miscolonization of the intestine.[52,57,58] In healthy persons, 20–30 g of undigested, fermentable carbohydrates will enter the large intestine every day. The stress limit for healthy persons is estimated at 20–50 g/day.[55] These and other scientific examinations suggest that fructose intolerance in a healthy adult is a normal phenomenon and that the tolerated amount of fructose is further reduced where there are general functional problems of the intestine and microbial miscolonization. According to this, fructose malabsorption in acquired secondary fructose intolerance is the result of damage to the small intestine's mucosa, caused by other diseases such as coeliac disease, acute gastrointestinal inflammation or Crohn's disease. Medicines, especially antibiotic therapy, can also be the source of the problem.
Similar to lactose malabsorption, fructose malabsorption leads to stomach aches, cramps, colics and flatulence due to fermentation gases, disintegrating, soft, often foul-smelling stool, diarrhoea, bloatedness or constipation. If fructose malabsorption persists, other, secondary symptoms will follow, caused by further resorption impairments (e.g. of the essential amino acid tryptophan, folic acid or zinc). Secondary symptoms are irritable bowel syndrome,[59] depression due to insufficient absorption[60] of the amino acid tryptophan (which is converted to serotonin and thus causes serotonin deficiency), fatigue,[58] headache,[54] nausea[54,58] and reflux.[58]
The hydrogen breathing tests for fructose

exposure and determination of the fructose level in the blood are also used for diagnosis. Acquired fructose malabsorption always coincides with bacterial miscolonization of the small intestine, since the change in intestinal flora reduces tolerance for fruit sugar.[61]

Histamine Intolerance

The cause of this impairment is acquired and arises from a lack of the enzymes diaminoxidase and histamine N-methyltransferase, which break down histamine. Histamine intolerance affects every hundredth person in Europe. Eighty percent of the cases are women.[62] Scientific indications for food intolerance due to biogenic amines such as histamine have not been documented yet.[46] Histamine intolerance is not considered a specific disease, but rather a side effect of other intolerances or allergies that cause this degradation impairment.

Histamine-containing foods
These foods include smoked meat, salami, ham, viscera, fish products and preserves, sea food, rope cheeses whose histamine content rises as the cheese matures, sauerkraut, spinach, beer, vinegar (and vinegar-containing products such as mustard or pickled vegetables), red wine and French champagne (because it contains red wine). Other foods include mushrooms and fungi in certain types of cheese, tomatoes, pizza, ketchup and chocolate. Pineapple, papayas, nuts and certain medicines further delay histamine degradation, and certain additives of the food industry increase the release of histamine in the body. If alcohol of any kind is drunk with histamine-containing food, severe reactions may occur because alcohol increases the permeability of the cell walls.

Medicines that may trigger reactions at histamine intolerance include analgesics and rheumatism medicines Mefenacid, Diclofenac and Indomethacin, and acetylic salicylic acid (aspirin). Fenbufen, Lefamisol and Ibuprofen are tolerated painkillers.

X-ray contrast agents will release histamine and may therefore be dangerous.

Typical symptoms of histamine intolerance occur after the corresponding triggers and include: headache, migraine, bronchial asthma, low blood pressure (hypotension), arrhythmia and menstruation problems (dysmenorrhoe). These symptoms do not prove histamine intolerance, since they can have various causes.

Diagnosis of histamine intolerance
The diagnosis is found by determining the histamine level and diaminoxydase in the blood, permitting only histamine-free food for two weeks and then measuring the same blood values. In case of histamine intolerance, the symptoms will improve considerably, the histamine level will drop by at least half and the level of the enzyme diaminoxydase will clearly increase. A provocation test with histamine would be too dangerous, since it may trigger life-threatening reactions.

For treatment of histamine intolerance, all histamine-containing food must be eliminated for the first two months. At the same time, the cause should be treated (i.e. healing of the miscolonization of the intestine) immediately, beginning with the fresh juice and almond milk diet of histamine-free fruits and vegetables; and after excluding milk protein allergy, with buttermilk, sour milk and a little quark and yoghurt. After two months, the blood values of histamine and diaminoxydase can be measured again. If they have normalised, the histamine-containing foods of raw vegetable food should be slowly reintroduced under observation, and one-third gently cooked vegetarian food can be added. Addition of vitamin B_6 also promotes the body's own synthesis of diaminoxydase.[63] Histamine intolerance heals hand in hand with the miscolonization of the small intestine (dysbiose).

The common cause and therapy of lactose, fructose and histamine intolerance

It has turned out that miscolonization of the intestine causes both acquired lactose and fructose intolerance, as well as hypersensitivity to histamine. These three conditions can be permanently healed by treating their shared cause. Widespread poor nutrition and the industrial processing of foods are the most important causes of miscolonization, and explain why these three problems have become common in our time. Today overly frequent antibiotic therapies also damage the ecosystem of the intestinal flora, sometimes massively.

The Problem of Food Allergy

The subject of food allergies is omnipresent. It is very important to differentiate between food intolerances and food allergies. A milk protein allergy to albumin or milk casein that can be documented with IgE is rare and severe, and yet more and more people tolerate milk and dairy products badly. This is because of the industrial processing of milk, homogenisation and UHT treatment. Fresh milk is treated at a pressure of 5 atm for homogenisation, so that the cream cannot precipitate anymore, and is sprayed onto a hot plate. This damages the spatial structure of the complex protein molecules and lipids. The enteral immune system reacts to this with suspicion and reduces tolerance, initially by producing IgG4-antibodies. People who have reacted with IgG4-antibodies to all dairy products in the lab test will in fact be unable to well tolerate pasteurised milk and Emmental cheese, while condensed milk will be tolerated easily. This contradicts the idea of milk protein allergy. A real milk protein allergy would cause an equal and severe reaction to all dairy products. Testing IgG4-antibodies against 260 foods will lead to a useful result regarding these sensitivities to many of the 260 foods. This procedure is very sensitive and must not be equated with an allergy. In our experience, the degree in which IgG4-antibodies for a certain food are present depends on the scope of the bacterial miscolonization, as well as the frequency at which it has been eaten. Additionally, we also observe cross-reactions to food that one has never or barely ever eaten. The IgG4-testing is a valuable help for planning the first diet steps for all disorders described in this book, almost all of which resulted from poor nutrition and a damaged micro flora (and its ultimate effects). In the scope of the forms of diet and diet stages listed in this book, it is worthwhile to leave out food (for 3–12 months, depending on the degree of reaction) for which high IgG4-antibody levels are present. These sensitivities usually disappear relatively quickly, so that they can gradually be reintroduced. Based on personal observation of food sensitivities in the body, many theories and nutrition teachings have emerged over the years without any scientific background at all. There are fashionable diets that appear quickly, confuse people and disappear again just as rapidly.

Crohn's disease

In 1904, the Polish surgeon Antoni Lesniowski first described this chronically inflammatory intestinal disease, named after the American doctor Burrill Bernard Crohn in 1932. The strange thing about this colitis is that, while it can occur in any section of the gastrointestinal tract, most frequently it is found in the ileum (i.e. the final section of the small intestine). Therefore it is also called Ileitis terminalis. What is even stranger is that this inflammation does not spread diffusely. It occurs very locally, and healthy mucosa sections alternate with very small affected areas, leading to a kind of 'cobblestone relief'. Therefore it is also called enteritis regionalis. Because the inflamed areas scar and harden, it is also called sclerosing chronic enteritis.

The number of persons suffering from Crohn's disease has increased steadily in recent years. In Western industrialised nations, 1–2 out of every thousand persons are affected by this severe disease, and at least 8 new cases per year occur per 100,000 persons. Crohn's disease usually affects young adults between 15 and 35 years of age, spread equally among women and men. It can also occur in persons aged 60 or older. Crohn's disease is a little more common among members of the same family.[64,65,66]

The cause of Crohn's disease has not been adequately established. B. B. Crohn believed that microbes in the intestinal mucosa cells caused the inflammation foci.
Current medical science classifies this disease as an autoimmune disease, because the inflammation symptoms can be suppressed by immunosuppression. Since this hypothesis states nothing about the cause, just as in the case of other autoimmune diseases, medical therapy remains a purely symptom-suppressing treatment and cannot heal the disease.[62,63] Only every fifth patient with Crohn's disease will show auto-antibodies (perinuclear anti-neutrophileous cytoplasmic antibodies, or p-ANCA). Failure of the congenital defence against intestinal bacteria is also held responsible for the inflammation.[67] Genetic examinations have provided little clarity regarding a genetic cause. Patients with Crohn's disease carry only three alleles (gene pairs) in chromosome 8 for the formation of β-defensins in the intestinal mucosa. These alleles act as natural antibiotics and lower β-defensin levels, but only if the disease occurs in the large intestine, rather than in the small intestine where the occurrence is much more frequent. In the affected small intestine, however, certain α-defensins of the affected mucosa are reduced, for which a mutation in gene NOD2/CARD15 that partially prevents the recognition of bacteria by the intestinal mucosa cells has been found. In spite of a certain frequency in families, a genetic cause of Crohn's disease has not yet been documented.[68]

In Crohn's disease, the tight junctions between the mucosa cells (enterocytes) are non-functional and reduced in number in the inflamed areas, so that toxic substances may pass through the mucosa. Epithelium cells die (apoptosis). There is a defect of the mucosa barrier, so that intestinal bacteria can enter the mucosa, which the immune system will counter with severe inflammation. This inflammation will damage the mucosa and its barrier function even more, thereby beginning a harmful, vicious circle. It is still quite unknown why it is possible for healthy mucosa islands to exist next to severely diseased spots.

People suffering from Crohn's disease suffer from iron deficiency. Ferroportin, a protein molecule, permits absorption of iron in the intestinal mucosa. This is inhibited by hepcidin, a substance in the intestine that prevents too much iron from entering the body. Crohn patients suffer from iron deficiency, since the production of hepcidin is strongly increased.

In two-thirds of the persons suffering from Crohn's disease, antibodies to the mycobacterium avium paratuberculosis can be found. In animals, this bacterium will produce chronic inflammation of the intestines. Paratuberculous cattle and Crohn patients share a defect in the gene CARD15/NOD2, which coincides with insufficient production of the natural intestinal antibiotic defensin in both. Mycobacterium avium paratuberculosis may cause inflammation of the intestines in humans.[69]

Crohn's disease is more common in areas with high standards of hygiene. It is suspected that soaps, softeners and emulsifiers may damage the mucosa barrier. This has not been proven, however.

The number of bacteria types in the intestinal flora is considerably reduced in Crohn patients. This shows that bacterial miscolonization of the small intestine plays a large part in the penetration of pathogenic bacteria and the barrier impairment in the affected intestinal sections. Persons suffering from Crohn's disease usually crave meat, tart, and spicy and fatty foods, and often reject fruit and raw vegetables. The stool is not only bloody but also slimy, explosive and of a foul odour. These are not only signs of inflammation of the intestines, but also of a generally massive miscolonization of the intestine. Putrefaction-producing anaerobic intestinal bacteria, such as clostridia, bacteroides, bifido bacteria, eubacteria, fusobacteria, ruminococci and roseburia, are part of the protein-induced flora of the large intestine. Anaerobic metabolism of proteins produces branched-chained fatty acids such as isovalerian acid, isobutyric acid, mercaptane, indole and toxic hydrogen sulphur gases that explain the manure-like or sulphur-like smell of the stool discharge. *Candida albicans* often grows well in the strongly impaired ecosystem of the intestinal flora in this disease. Its degradation products may cause neurogenic amines with an adrenaline-line effect. When this is the case, the patients suffer from stress symptoms such as anxiety, heat and tachycardia.

The regulation of the autonomous nervous system is usually overexcited (hypersympathicotonie). Crohn's disease is also called a psychosomatic condition because stress, fear or mental trauma may trigger a new episode.

In our experience, Crohn's disease is the consequence of a massively impaired life order and poor nutrition, where massive microbial imbalance (dysbiosis) with toxic intestinal putrefaction has damaged the mucosa barrier of the intestine. The ileum is directly in front of the large intestine and most exposed to the entry of anaerobic, putrefaction-producing large-intestine bacteria. Therefore the ileum is usually affected by Crohn's disease. Mucosa areas that resist the toxin effect the least will suffer massive infection, with penetration of toxin-forming bacteria and toxins and destruction of the enterocytes (apoptosis). The inflammation penetrates the mucosa and the vascular and muscle-containing layers of the intestinal wall, resulting in massive bleeding, cramps or sharp pain.

The pain occurs very often in the lower-right abdomen (ileum), often after eating. However, it may also occur in other intestinal segments. The inflammation leads to a severe diarrhoea-like discharge, the attempt of the intestine to expel the toxins – sometimes imperatively and explosively, often violently – up to 10 times per day. Fever, appetite and loss of weight are the rule during the episodes, often accompanied by nausea and vomiting. In spite of immunosuppressive treatment, the episodes often last for weeks, requiring inpatient treatment. Anaemia, iron deficiency and vitamin-B_{12} deficiency (if the ileum is affected) are the rule and must be corrected.

Half of the patients suffering from Crohn's disease also suffer from general symptoms caused by toxins and metabolites in the inflamed intestine. These include joint pain, arthritis, rashes such as erythema nodosum (areas with nodular inflamed swelling), putrid gangrene (pyoderma gangraenosum) or rosacea. The iris of the eyes is often inflamed as well (uveitis). In a few patients, these extra-intestinal symptoms occur years before the inflammation of the intestines occurs. Additionally, patients suffer from the numerous side effects of the symptom-suppressing medication.

Inflammation episodes may also lead to complications. During the course of the disease, 20–30 % of all patients suffer from ileus. Initially this is caused by swelling of the inflamed section, and later by scar structures. In addition, fistulas often form. Fistulas are open connections between the intestine and the body surface, the vagina and the skin next to the anus. Less frequently, pus collections will encapsulate (abscesses) or inflammation toxins will cause massive, slack expansion of the large intestine (toxic megacolon). A colonoscopy should be performed at least once a year because of the risk of malignant mutation of chronically inflamed areas (carcinoma of the small intestine). Many patients suffer from osteoporosis as a result of malabsorption, particularly as a side effect of cortisol medication. Gall stones result from overloaded enterohepatic circulation and oxalate kidney stones because the ileum can no longer properly absorb bile acids, which remove calcium from the oxalic acid.

Every first intestinal bleeding requires a careful examination of the intestine. The typical 'cobblestone relief' and histology (tissue microscopy) permit diagnosis.

Treatment for Crohn's Disease
Medication for suppressing symptoms is differentiated into *episode treatment* and *remission treatment* between the episodes, and aims to reduce the frequency of episodes. Surgical removal of the affected intestinal sections is avoided where possible, since new sections of the intestine will probably be affected afterwards. The procedure has been established in European regulations.[70]

Medical treatment of acute episodes
During an acute episode, academic medicine requires either a synthetic, fully re-absorbable fibre-rich liquid diet through a gastric tube, or parenteral nutrition via infusions. Synthetic adrenal hormones (cortisol) such as prednisone are highly dosed to suppress the immune response to toxic cell damage. In nine out of ten patients, a high dose of prednisone is enough to suppress the current episode. If the inflammation is located in the ileum or the right large intestine, the steroid preparation budesonide is often used for its particularly strong effects in the ileum and right large intestine. If the rectum is affected, cortisol can be used as an enema. If the episode is located in the left large intestine and not too strong, salazosulfapyridin, a salicylic acid, or mesazalin may also slightly reduce inflammation.

The suppressing effect of these medicines will make the disease chronic, so that the dosages must be increased at regular intervals. When cortisol becomes ineffective, the immunosuppressants infliximab or adalimumab (called tumour necrosis factor blockers, or TNF-blockers) are used. These have severe side effects.

Medication for remission treatment
There is still no medication that can prevent acute episodes of Crohn's disease. First, academic medicine utilizes mainly the immune-suppressants azathioprine, 6-mercaptopurin and methotrexate. This therapy accepts the risks of severe side effects, which must be recognised early in narrow lab examinations.
Second, once these immune-suppressants are no longer sufficient, formation inhibitors of the tumour necrosis factor α will be used (TNF-α-blockers): infliximab, adalimumab or, in Switzerland, certolizumab.

Chronic infections may increase due to this (e.g. in case of scarred tuberculosis). Third, integrin antagonists are used: vedolizumab. These medicines may have dangerous side effects.

Malabsorption puts patients at risk of nutrient deficiencies, especially iron, vitamin B_{12}, zinc and selenium. Patients may also suffer from osteoporosis as a side effect of cortisol.

The dietetic causal treatment

In our experience, Crohn's disease can be healed by consistent dietetic treatment of the cause of the disease, the nutritional deficiency of the intestinal flora and overgrowth of the small intestine with anaerobic, toxin-forming large-intestinal bacteria, or intestinal putrefaction. Many foods, even healthful ones, are not tolerated at first in many cases because their nutrients have passed through the defective mucosa barrier for years, triggering allergic reactions. An allergological examination of IgE-antibodies in the blood is not sensitive enough.

By contrast, analysis of the IgG4-antibodies in the serum against all important foods is very helpful. If apples are tolerated, it is sensible to start with hydrocolon therapy and an apple diet week, and then to proceed with a broken-down raw food diet in the form of fresh juices from foods that are both allergologically tolerated and intestine calming (see table). Almond milk should be taken with every fresh juice meal.

Chronic inflammation, pain, oxidative stress and anaemia often leave patients exhausted at first. This state can be reliably relieved by mitochondrial-infusion therapy with glutathione-vitamin C infusions, procain-base infusions, and coenzyme Q-10, in addition to the regenerating effect of the diet. Mitochondria, the 'power plants' of the cells which produce the energy-rich phosphates for cell metabolism by glucose breakdown, regenerate under this therapy and will reproduce again. This means that the cell energy will improve relatively quickly. Deficiencies in iron, vitamin B_{12}, zinc or selenium must be quickly corrected.

Every patient requires a customized diet plan. Fructose intolerance may be present. In that case, vegetable instead of fruit juices must be used at first, with vegetables which contain as little fructose as possible. After testing for milk protein tolerance, several days of the sour milk diet are required. If desired, buttermilk may be added to the almond milk to support the fermenting of facultative anaerobic bacteria that should dominate in the small intestine and that have lost their 'home rights' against the immigrated anaerobic large-intestinal bacteria, the enterococci and lacto bacillus types. This procedure may settle healthy small-intestinal bacteria and drive the pathogenic immigrated anaerobes of the large intestine out of the small intestine.

Suspensions with autolysed healthy intestinal bacteria may improve the immune tolerance of the intestine for germs to be settled, so that they can develop better (symbiosis control). Soon the raw food diet can be begun. Preference should be given to food with secondary plant substances that have an anti-inflammatory and anti-infectious effect. Fresh fruit and vegetables have an anti-inflammatory effect and will soon be tolerated. Apples, bananas, blueberries, beetroots, blackberries, dark cherries, mangoes, pomegranates and tomatoes are particularly suitable. Once the diarrhoea has largely subsided, this diet can be sharply enhanced. After a few weeks, one-third gently cooked vegan food can be added to what is already tolerated.

Therapy of the cause will require complete information and consistent cooperation of the patient. The immunosuppressive therapy can be reduced step by step, and the dosage of cortisol can be very slowly reduced to a small maintenance dose of 5–10 mg of prednisone/day, since pain episodes with bleeding will abate. The formation of natural cortisol in the adrenal cortex will have been suppressed by several years of prednisone, and the adrenal cortex will be atrophied. Therefore the last dose of prednisone can usually be discontinued only after the disease has been healed completely. The adrenal cortex must regenerate and relearn to produce a normal, healthy cortisol level. During the first months of this therapy, episodes will recur. However, they will soon be much weaker and will slowly decrease in frequency. During an episode, neural therapy can be a great help by treating the coeliac ganglia, as well as local treatment of the inflamed intestinal section. This usually makes it possible to stop pain and bleeding immediately. Fungal infestation with *Candida albicans* cannot be removed by antibiotic treatment, but will disappear within a few weeks or months under the above dietetic treatment, since the fungi will be displaced by the newly settled healthy small-intestinal bacteria. This will treat the overexcitation of the vegetative nervous system, which has been caused by the metabolites of the *Candida* fungi.

Crohn's disease cannot be healed solely by homoeopathy, which is unable to change the intestinal milieu. However, the information of a homoeopathic treatment coordinated precisely with the symptoms, modalities, constitutional features and mental situation of the patient may support healing. Homoeopathy is not a placebo therapy but a pharmacological information therapy. It is not the substance but the information stored in it that acts on the biological system by deleting false information, similar to informatics, where a program loaded onto a CD can re-order a damaged programme. Homoeopathic treatment requires considerable knowledge and experience. It must be handled by a specialist. Properly chosen, the homoeopathic medication has a very quick and clearly noticeable effect. If nothing changes for a long time, the treatment was wrong. To risk overreactions, one starts with the first Q-potency and increases slowly.

Treatment of Crohn's disease requires a doctor and demands great experience and knowledge. It is then a thankful and fascinating task for the doctor and his patient – a task that will be worth the effort

Colitis Ulcerosa

In industrialised Western countries, approx. every 500th person contracts this inflammatory, bleeding intestinal disease. Each year 3–7 new cases are counted per 100,000 persons. Women and men are equally affected. Colitis ulcerosa used to be rare even in industrialised Western countries but has grown in frequency in recent decades. Is used also to be rare in Africa, Asia and South America. Increasing industrialisation, changes in lifestyle and nutritional habits, and the increasingly large offer of industrially processed foods have made this disease increasingly common in these countries.

Colitis ulcerosa affects only the large intestine. Large areas of the mucosa become inflamed and are destroyed. Since the inflammation forms ulcers (ulcerosa) and penetrates into deeper, vasculated layers, the patient will lose a significant amount of blood.

The cause of colitis ulcerosa is unknown. As in Crohn's disease, the NF-κB-transcription factor is suspected, but a genetic cause has not really been proven. As in Crohn's disease, higher hygiene standards, with the use of numerous detergents and emulsifiers that may enter the intestine, are suspected of being a contributing factor in colitis ulcerosa. However, in addition to higher hygiene standards, the industrialised states of the 'civilised world' have seen an enormous increase of generally poor nutrition, industrial processing of food with its innumerable flavours, preservatives and additives, and consumption of industrially processed products. People who have been treated with antibiotics repeatedly or for long periods – particularly in childhood – will more frequently suffer from colitis ulcerosa later in life. As in Crohn's disease, this suggests a great importance of damaged intestinal flora with miscolonization by pathogenic germs as causes of colitis ulcerosa and Crohn's disease. The scientifically confirmed positive effect of the probiotic Mutaflor, a medicine with the healthy population of living bacteria of Escherichia coli of the species Nissle 1917, suggests this.[70, 71]

Like Crohn's disease, colitis ulcerosa comes in episodes that can be triggered by stress and mental strain. The episodes produce massive, slimy, bloody diarrhoea and very painful colic. The patients are very stressed by the frequency of defecation and the unexpectedly sudden character with explosive discharge, and may find themselves in impossible situations where they cannot retain their stool. They are physically debilitated and emaciated. Sugar-containing food (fructose, lactose, sorbite) causes painful flatulence crises (secondary fructose and lactose intolerance).

About one-fifth of the patients with ulcerous colitis suffer from symptoms outside of the digestive tract, as in Crohn's disease. About 10 % suffer from ankylosing spondylitis which, similar to Bechterev's disease, causes the longitudinal ligaments of the spine to become painfully inflamed. Every fourth patient develops a very painful inflammation of the sacroiliac joint (sacroileitis). Of all patients, 11 % develop painful inflammation (arthritis) that occurs in several joints, about 17 % develop nodular inflammation foci in the skin (erythema nodosum), and 1 % suffer from the ulcerous putrid Pyoderma gangrenosum of the skin. Approx. 3 % of all patients suffering from colitis ulcerosa also suffer from very painful inflammation of the outer skin of the eyes (episcleritis) or uveitis, inflammation of the iris; and 7 % suffer from scarring bile duct inflammation (primary sclerosing cholangitis). Every other colitis-ulcerosa patient will suffer from bone loss, which turns into manifest osteoporosis in every seventh patient.

In the acute episode, 40 bloody stool discharges per day under pain and fever are not rare. Urination may be painful as well. Weight loss, utter exhaustion and anaemia with tachycardia torment the patients.
The toxins of pathogenic intestinal bacteria and disintegrating substances from the inflammation foci in the large intestine often cause the large intestine to soften and become slack and expanded during the episodes (toxic megacolon), and the peritoneum becomes inflamed. Perforations of the large intestine into the abdominal cavity occur and are very dangerous.
The inflamed mucosa forms polyps that may mutate into cancer of the large intestine after eight to ten years of illness. Therefore, an annual colonoscopy must be recommended after more than eight years of illness, to find any tumours as early as possible. After ten years of disease, 2.1 % of all patients suffer from colon carcinoma (cancer of the large intestine). After 20 years this number grows to 8.5 %, and after 30 years the number grows to 17.8 %.

Suppression medication
This is specified in the European directives.[71] Because medications do not tackle

the cause, but merely suppress inflammation (and thus symptoms), they promote chronicity of the condition and slowly lose their effectiveness. The result is that increasingly high doses and additional immunosuppressive medication will be required to treat the episodes.

Therapy during the acute episode
Cortisol is given at high dosage during the episode, as an infusion or as prednisone tablets, until the bleeding stops. These steroid hormones can then be reduced gradually by the doctor while the patient is closely monitored. Fluid and blood loss and shifts in the electrolyte and trace-element balance – especially of sodium, magnesium, zinc and selenium – must be monitored and corrected. Anaemia and iron deficiencies must be corrected and vitamin levels must be monitored.
Steroid hormones (cortisol) are not always enough to suppress an episode. In such cases, the immune-suppressants and anti-metabolites described below will be added step by step and as required.

Permanent therapy
When the episode has subsided, permanent therapy will follow with the target of delaying and weakening further episodes. Mesazalin is recommended for permanent therapy, since it inhibits inflammation and seems to slightly reduce cancer risk. Mesazalin inhibits folic-acid absorption, so the folic-acid level must be monitored. If mesazalin is not tolerated, sulfasalazine can be administered. If this is still not enough, cortisol is applied locally as budesonide foam or an enema. Mesazalin can also be administered to the rectum as a suppository, enema or foam. If this is still not enough, the dosage of the cortisol (i.e. the prednisone tablets) will be increased. Mutaflor consists of bacteria of the species *Escherichia coli* Nissle 1917. Several studies have documented that Mutaflor is more effective against colitis episodes than is mesazalin.[72,73] If the immune suppression must be increased, azathioprine will also be administered. If it is not tolerated, 6-mercaptopurin is used. If this is still not enough, the anti-metabolites methotrexate, cyclosporine or tacrolimus will be used. If this still is not enough, blockers of the cytokine tumour necrosis factor α (TNF-blockers) with their many side effects will be used, among them the drug infliximab. In the excessive rush of pharma-industrial competition, more and more immunosuppressive medicines are coming onto the market. All of them are very expensive and some can have dangerous side effects.

Surgical therapy
If after several years none of this has helped, the official treatment directives recommend amputation of the diseased organ, i.e. surgical removal of the entire large intestine and rectum. To collect stool before discharge, a loop of the small intestine will be used to fashion a bag (j-pouch), a newly produced reservoir situated near where the rectum would normally be. Now the diseased organ is removed and can no longer become inflamed. These patients often suffer from stool incontinence, however, as well as from inflammations of the artificial anus or erectile dysfunction (impotence).

Medication of complementary medicine
For thousands of years, myrrh has proven its worth as a herb against inflammations. The first scientific investigations of its effectiveness in colitis ulcerosa have already been performed.[74] Myrrh relaxes the muscles of the intestinal walls and is supposed to relieve tenesmus and cramps cause by this disease. A randomised double-blind study showed that myrrh combined with chamomile and coffee coal has the same degree of effect as mesazalin.[75] Frankincense (Boswellia serrata), a very old healing herb, contains inflammation-

inhibiting bosweila acids that can offer relief in inflammatory intestinal diseases such as colitis ulcerosa.[76] The lecithin content in the intestine of patients with colitis ulcerosa is much reduced. Lecithin is very important for the mucosa barrier in the intestine and to prevent entry of bacteria and toxins into the intestinal walls. Lecithin is available in a galenic form that enters the large intestine undigested. It is to improve the mucosa barrier and thus also relieve inflammation. The effect of lecithin in colitis ulcerosa is currently undergoing scientific examination. Liquorice, as succus liquiriziae, has an anti-inflammatory effect on mucosae. Liquorice can be used as a rinsing enema, and better yet as retention enemas to reduce colitis.[77] These rinses should be alternated with chamomile and astringent phytotherapeutics such as tormentilla and tannin-containing plants (e.g. anserines and tormentilla), as well as with enemas using St. John's wort, which promotes wound-healing.[75]

The therapy of colitis ulcerosa is satisfactory for neither patients nor attending doctors. It reflects the powerlessness of our modern medical science against this disease. It calls for new insights – a new, entirely different understanding of the causes and the development of the disease.

Dietary Treatment of Colitis Ulcerosa
In our experience, just as in Crohn's disease, there is significant miscolonization of the intestine at the cause of this condition, where the toxin-forming intestinal bacteria dominate and attack and destroy the intestinal mucosa with their toxins. This disease also causes the barrier function of the intestinal wall to be broken, so that the immune system will react with massive defence against the entering substances from the intestinal contents and the bacteria toxins and against substances from degenerated or already destroyed intestinal mucosa cells, starting a vicious circle of destructive inflammation.

Our dietetic treatment of colitis ulcerosa is, as for Crohn's disease, designed to restore the massively damaged ecosystem of the intestinal flora and to ensure energetic and substance nutrition of the intestinal mucosa cells. The dietetic procedure is described in detail in this book for the therapy of Crohn's disease, with dietary specifications and tables. It can be read and applied in close cooperation with the attending physician, under individual adjustment to the condition of the patient and tested food allergies and intolerances. With long-term, consistent execution of these dietary provisions, this therapy will have a reliable effect, so that the symptom-suppressing therapy can be slowly reduced. Much later, after complete healing, when episodes no longer occur with the minimum dosage of prednisone, this small remaining dosage can be given every other day, and later every third day. This alternating procedure will allow the adrenal cortex to regenerate and relearn to produce a normal, natural cortisol level which, for all healthy persons, is required physiologically and to maintain health. If the alternating dosage does not trigger any symptoms, the medication can be discontinued.
In our experience, colitis ulcerosa usually heals faster than Crohn's disease. It is very important that our vital vegetable-based diet be followed throughout the patient's life, after this severe disease of the large intestine has healed. Under these conditions, recurrences are not expected. It is a path that is worth the effort.

Diverticular Disease (Diverticulosis)

Diverticula are small bulges of the large intestine's mucosa. A small weak spot in the intestinal wall causes the intestinal mucosa to bulge outward like a small bag. In industrialised Western countries, more than half of all persons aged above 60 suffer from diverticula, which will be found during a colonoscopy and will usually not cause any problems.

Symptoms occur when one or several of these diverticula become inflamed (diverticulitis). Treated with antibiotics, the symptoms will usually recur soon and become more and more frequent, until the affected intestinal segment scars, stiffens and narrows. From the second inflammation period onwards, academic medicine recommends that the affected part of the intestine be removed.

Inflamed diverticula may burst and discharge into the abdominal cavity. Less frequently, they burst into another organ, such as the vagina or the bladder, leading to an abnormal connection called a fistula. Stool will then discharge from the vagina or the bladder will become massively infected. Another complication is diverticulum bleeding, which is one of the most common causes of intestinal bleeding in older persons. The affected segment of the large intestine then must be removed by emergency surgery.
Usually the rectum is affected by diverticulitis. This is then usually possible with endoscopic surgery, and an artificial bowel outlet will not be necessary.

Diverticulosis and diverticulitis occur in the intestines of those persons who eat low fibre food, large quantities of animal protein, fat and food prepared with white flour. In their intestines, putrefaction-producing anaerobic bacteria dominate and form toxic flatulence gases.
This disease is prevented by nutrition with mostly vegetable-based fresh food.

In the case of diverticulitis, neural therapy can usually stop the inflammation immediately and thus prevent surgery. We treat the affected intestinal segment as well as the sympathetic trunk. During this and on subsequent days, the patient must be monitored closely by a doctor. The nutrition must then be changed thoroughly in order to prevent relapses.

Cancer of the Large Intestine (Colon Carcinoma)

Frequency
More than 95 % of all malignant tumours of the intestine occur in the large intestine. In western European countries, the frequency of intestinal cancers has doubled in the last 30 years, from 20 to 40 new cases per 100,000 residents. Today more than 6 % of Germans contract colorectal carcinoma in the course of their lives, and 3 % die from this disease,[78] the second most common cancer. Sixty percent of all patients are men and forty percent are women. Nine out of ten new cases occur in persons older than 50. Three hundred out of every 1,000 persons aged 45–75 have colon polyps, and 10 suffer from undetected cancer of the large intestine.[79]
This cancer almost always grows from benign polyps of the large intestine's mucosa. Eight out of ten of these tumours result from the genetic mutation of a glandular cell (adenocarcinoma). Sixty percent of the tumours occur in the left part of the large intestine and 25 % in the caecum and the right large intestine. About half of the left part intestine tumours occur in the sigmoid loop, the S-shaped connection between the descending large intestine and the rectum and in the rectum itself.

Prevention of cancer of the large intestine
Smoking increases almost all cancer risks massively, including that of colon cancer.[80] Obesity increases the risk of cancer of the large intestine.[81,59,97] It declines signifi-

cantly with increased physical activity.[82,83,96] The daily ingestion of red meat (pork or beef), meat products and sausages increases the risk of colon cancer by more than 50 %, while fish instead of meat reduces it.[84] Low-fibre nutrition with large quantities of carbohydrates such as sugar and white flour foods increases the risk of colon cancer.[85] Increased intake of fibre reduces the risk of cancer of the large intestine by 40 %.[86, 20] Bile acids are chemically converted by the bacteria of the intestinal flora into secondary bile acid (desoxycholic acid and lithocholic acid). They cause cancer in the large intestine.[87] They are bound by ballasts, so that nutrition with abundant fruit, vegetables, salads and whole cereals also protects from cancer because of its high fibre content.[88] When the fibre is broken down by bacteria, short chain fatty acids are produced in the intestine. Among the fatty acids, butyric acid particularly protects from cancer. Butyric acid inhibits the cell division activity of the cells of the large intestine's mucosa and increases the degree of their differentiation into healthy cells.[89] Regular consumption of apple juice helps prevent cancer of the large intestine.[90,91]

As it occurs in fruit and vegetables, β-carotene reduces cancer risk in the large intestine by 44 %.[92] Foods that protect from cancer are: broccoli, green cabbage, carrots, tomatoes, whole wheat, whole barley, fresh soy beans, apricots, lemons, garlic, onions and flaxseeds. All should be eaten raw, if possible.[93] All other vegetables and fruits have a weaker but still decisive effect on cancer.[90] Most vegetable substances that protect from cancer also effectively fight existing tumours.[90, 94] As part of raw food therapy against cancer, they should be used intensely in the regime. Cooking will destroy more than half of the anti-carcinogenic effect of raw vegetable food, which should be eaten mainly raw when cancer is present.[90] Family members of patients suffering from cancer of the large intestine will develop the same kind of cancer about three times more often than normal. This does not prove that they are genetically more at risk. Rather, they usually have similar eating habits. Persons with colitis ulcerosa or Crohn's disease develop colon cancer about three times more often, as mentioned above.[95,96] There are eight different genetic peculiarities in which cancer of the large intestine is particularly common, affecting 8 % of new cases. Not all of these patients have colon polyps.

The symptoms of cancer of the large intestine
Early recognition is very difficult because this cancer can progress without symptoms for a long time. Blood in the stool is a typical early symptom. The cause must be found at once. Later, stool habits will change, and much later there will be uncharacteristic stomach ache or cramps. Even later, ileus will force the patient to the emergency ward.

Therapy and prognosis
In the early stages, when the cancer has only affected the mucosa (and particularly if it has grown into the intestine, as polyps), the cancer can be healed through small abdominal cuts by the microsurgical removal of the affected intestinal segment with its lymph nodes. If these lymph nodes contain cancer cells, chemotherapy is recommended afterwards. Usually a stoma can be avoided.

If the tumour is located in the rectum, radiation is usually recommended before surgery. If it is only in the mucosa, it can be removed through the anus. If it goes more deeply, it must be removed with a significant quantity of surrounding tissue. An artificial bowel outlet is usually required, at least temporarily.

If the cancer has grown deeper into

healthy tissues or has already formed metastases, major surgery is required, usually after prior treatment with chemotherapy.

Prognosis in the case of cancer of the large intestine

If the tumour is limited to the mucosae, the patients will remain healthy for more than five years. Recurrences after this are rare. If the tumour has grown into the lymph nodes, four out of ten patients will remain without recurrence for five years; after remote metastases, 20 % of all patients will remain without recurrence. Chemotherapy is better tolerated with a concurrent raw food diet.[97,98,99,100] Wound healing is also improved by this diet. Scientific insights so far have confirmed the hypothesis that dietetic therapy of the cause reduces the risk of a tumour recurrence and later formation of metastases. Therefore we recommend starting it at once, in all cases.

Dr. med. Maximilian Bircher-Benner was invited in 1937 to give a lecture cycle at the University of Oxford by Prof. McCarrison. A short time later Dr. med. Maximilian Bircher-Benner repeated the lecture in Zurich, in the auditorium of the ETH ZURICH, the university for science and technology,.[101] After lifelong experience in the treatment of many thousands of patients at his hospital, including cancer patients, and decades of clinical dietetic research of this phenomenon, he said the following:

'Millions have been spent on cancer research. Hecatombs of animals had to be experimented on. Little was gained from this. The researchers are still not clear about the causes of cancer. In Philadelphia, a great book by the renowned cancer researcher Frederick L. Hoffmann has just been published, with the simple title: *Cancer and Nutrition*.[102] In this work a huge number of facts and observations have been collected that suggest that 1) cancer is a disease of the entire organism, and 2) pervasive nutritional influences are to be considered causative factors.

'All in all, Hoffmann believes that "too much food" is a cause of cancer. The core of the matter is what is hidden behind this "too much". Hoffmann's statistical research is still weak here. If you have become familiar with the effect of food on the human organism in long research and medical life, as *Hindhede* and *McCarrison*, myself and others have, you will see cancer as the product of long term disorderly nutrition, encouraged by other disorders in life.

'The only great experiment that would make this clear – *Rollo Rüssel* suggested it 25 years ago – has not been started yet. It would require a few thousand properly informed persons to eat in an ordered way throughout their lives, permitting comparison of the numbers of cancers between them and the overall population, to demonstrate a great difference to their benefit. Since the so-called healthy person does not want to hear anything about changing his life habits, persuasion must be applied to the tired, ill person, and through him to his family. My experience shows that this path is successful. My suggestion therefore is not to spend millions on animal experiments, but millions on public health centres with order therapy. This is the path towards mastering the disease of cancer, that terrible plague.

'Ladies and gentlemen! You can see that man must pay for life in the realm of disorder into which he has unwittingly ventured, with an immense amount of illness, disease, suffering, pain and distress. Is this not all hell on earth? Is it not time to finally think of returning to the realm of order?'

These were the words with which Bircher-Benner ended his second lecture. Since then there have been many epidemiological research results and fascinating scientific insights from basic research that have begun consistently to create a picture of the causes of cancer and most chronic diseases, as with pieces of a mosaic. It is not necessary to wait for a conclusion. There are enough insights to begin dietetic prophylaxis and support the dietetic therapy of cancer.

The Effect of Food on the Digestive Tract

Two types of food energy

Physicists are aware of two types of energy: the orderly and the chaotic. Orderly energy saves information. Chaotic energy cannot save anything. Heat energy is chaotic energy. Sunlight is the most highly ordered type of energy. Its information is similar to a large symphony. Listening to a symphony does not produce heat, but it provides information: a highly orderly sound structure that triggers precise sensations and feelings. With its complex oscillations, sunlight conveys and orders the genetically specific information that is needed for growth, differentiation and regeneration of all life on earth.

One green leaf contains about one million chlorophyll funnels. At the base of each funnel, there are two chlorophyll α molecules. The funnel reflects the incoming light into the base, where the chlorophyll α molecules enter into maximum resonance, synchronised with the oscillations of the solar radiation (coherence). They convert the energy from this resonance into UV light, which makes them light up (invisibly to our eyes). This light flows through the entire plant body all the way into the tips of the roots.[103] All living cells store UV light in their molecules, and particularly in the ring-shaped molecules. The double helix of the genetic material in the cell cores stores the most light by far. The double helix (DNA) can coil to the right or left and can form protrusions shaped like clover leaves, radiating specific UV light spectrums.[104] The double helix of the DNA serves as a cavity resonator for the rhythmic laser amplification of UV light in our cells.[105] For a laser to begin to work, it must receive a certain amount of energy. Bio-physicians call this minimum energy supply the laser threshold. In their experiments, researchers of the international academy for bio-photon research measured the laser threshold in plant tissues.[100, 101, 106]

Just like plants, human and animal cells store UV light in their DNA.[99, 101] However, we lack the ability to photosynthesise, and direct application of sunlight to the skin is not nearly enough to keep our laser-light storage above the laser threshold.

The plant's cell stores the photons from sunlight in extremely large amounts. It could be shown that ultra-weak cell radiation[107] is nothing but a kind of leakage radiation, a tiny leak of the UV-light through the cell membrane. Measurements have shown that laser amplification of the light is 10^4 times stronger in the DNA than that provided by technical laser devices. The inside of the cells is thus an incredible light space. Our photon store must be provisioned daily with a sufficient amount of living photon-containing foods (fresh vegetables).[108,109,102]

The transmission of the information contained in the cellular UV light from photosynthesis in living foods to our organism takes place by coherence. This means that our own sensation of life, our life energy and life information, is repeatedly renewed and reordered in the roughly 15 trillion cells of our body by entering into a shared resonance with the oscillation patterns of sunlight upon transfer of the photons.

If living foods are missing from our nutrition, the photon content in our cells will decline. The light content will decrease until it falls below the laser threshold. The consequence is degeneration.

Dr. med. Maximilian Bircher-Benner explained the amazing effect of his diet by the second main principle of thermodynamics, the law of entropy, based on his scientific research over several years.[105] In fact, it is surprising that our modern medical sciences still use calories and calorific values as the only measure for food energy, while the second main principle of thermodynamics has been the basis for all energy considerations in all other scientific areas, in technology, physics and chemistry for 150 years.

In the early 20th century, the fear of infection by bacteria ruled the medical world. The belief that all food ought to be cooked before eating led to new demands for the hygienic preparation of raw vegetables. When heat-sensitive vitamins and vital substances were discovered, Bircher-Benner's raw food diet set out on its way to global recognition.

Research into the laser amplification of photons in the genetic material of living cells,[99,100,101,102] and into information transmission and storage in the basic substance of the connective tissue,[110] confirms Bircher-Benner's hypothesis of light accumulation in living foods and the enormous importance of photosynthesis for the energy value of foods as ordering and thus healing information for the biological system of the human being.

Further confirmation from basic research came in the papers of Nobel Prize Laureate Ilya Prigogine[111] on the dissipative system of living cells, which showed that the striving of all physical processes for disorder (law of entropy) does not apply to living cells, since the storage of photons from photosynthesis and the enormous rhythmical reinforcement of this light in the cells according to the laser principle removes them from the thermodynamic balance, to the extent that the second main principle of energetics does not apply and the chaos principle turns into an ordering coherence principle.

In fact, all the living cells of nature are the only place where small, simple molecules are turned into complex, high order molecules, processes and structures: where chaos becomes order. This is what makes the raw food diet so important as the only regime that transfers the ordering principle and effect of living cells to our biological system and thus produces its great ordering and healing effect.

Furthermore, fresh vegetable food offers high nutritional economy,[94, 97] in which all nutrients are organically bound at suitable ratios and thus become highly available biologically. Fresh vegetable food also provides the enzymes required for the assimilation of living substances, as well as a high content of polyphenols, carotenes and other antioxidants which have a powerful protective effect from degeneration and genetic mutation, and thus from cancer.

Furthermore, there is the great regulating effect that raw food has on the ecosystem of the bacteria flora of the intestine, so that infections, excessive fermentation or intestinal putrefaction, and cancer can be prevented.

The pure raw food diet, when administered by a qualified professional, is the ideal healing regime to prevent and heal any degenerative disease of the kind described as 'civilisation diseases', which have spread continuously in our time. It is a path that is worth the effort.

General Guidelines for Treatment of Intestinal Diseases

For practical instructions, consult the chapter on Forms of Diet, tables I and II and the recipe section.

Three forms of diet have proven their worth in treating intestinal disease:

The Raw Apple Diet (Especially in Case of Diarrhoea)

One to two kilograms of grated apples per day. The grated apples should be very fresh at all times (they must not turn brown). The low protein content of this diet withdraws nutrition from the protein-consuming, putrefaction-producing bacteria. The fruit acids inhibit growth of these putrefaction pathogens. The pectin content of the apples absorbs the harmful bacterial disintegration products (toxins), thus preventing them from entering the body through the mucosa.

The Raw Food Diet

The carotenoids, especially the beta carotene of the fruits and vegetables, stimulate the reproduction of monocytes and macrophages (scavenger cells), the formation of cytosines, tumour necrosis factor α (which is also important for protecting from infection), and interleukin 1β. Beta carotene also increases the natural killer cells circulating in the blood. Vitamin A stimulates the immune system, as does the vitamin C from fruits. The flavonoids of the fruits modulate the immune system to dampen and inhibit the inflammatory reaction, and also partially inhibit prostaglandin formation. All of these secondary plant substances modulate the immune system in the desired direction.

Secondary plant substances in fresh fruit and vegetables also have an antibiotic effect.

Vegetables with a particularly strong antibiotic effect may not be used while the intestine is irritated, since some of them would further irritate the mucosa. These include garlic, cress, mustard, horseradish, raw whole wheat and tomatoes. However, they may be used after conditions have calmed and after careful testing of compatibility. Raw fresh fruit and vegetable food has the highest potential of highly ordered, biologically available energy from sunlight and the sunlight's content in ordering and thus healing biological information. Raw food regulates the ecosystem of the intestinal flora reliably back to its healthy balance, so that putrefaction-producing protein-consuming bacteria that form toxic gases (e.g. methane and hydrogen sulphur) are displaced to the benefit of healthy intestinal bacteria. The raw food diet also reliably overcomes the laziness of the intestine, so that healthy peristalsis will slowly return to being predominant. The diet is composed economically, in the sense that the digestive system and the metabolism will not be stressed with useless substances and their metabolites, and will be able to recover. Thus the enterohepatic circulation (i.e. excessive circulation of the products of food-degradation between the intestine and liver through the portal system) is also massively relieved, so that the intestine and liver can both recover. For gastrointestinal diseases, food and its mechanical preparation must be carefully adjusted to the condition of the patient, and administered in the form of fresh juices, purees or finely chopped ingredients, with nut or almond milk (see tables).

The Sour Milk Diet

Milk-protein allergies were rare 40 years ago. However, infant formula and the industrial processing of cow milk before it even appears in the stores have increased the frequency of milk intolerance. For homogenisation, milk is pressurised at 5 atm and sprayed onto a hot plate. This cripples the spatial structure of the large molecules and prevents the milk from turning into cream. Molecules modified in this manner will be perceived by the immune system of the intestine as suspicious proteins. The immune system triggers defensive reactions. A sour milk diet is a good way of regulating the intestinal flora, but must only be used if milk protein is tolerated. The sour milk products must not have been pasteurised.

A sour milk diet with buttermilk and yoghurt contains lacto bacilli and other bifidus bacteria. They promote healthy germs in the intestine and displace the putrefaction bacteria that form toxic methane and hydrogen sulphur. The sour milk diet helps to acidulate the intestinal flora so that healthy bacteria flourish. This diet form is particularly suitable for persons with constipation, putrefaction, dyspepsia and flatulence (meteorism) and may also be used temporarily with professional support in cases of chronic colitis. Pure lactic acid, applied in a highly diluted form, may in some cases have a beneficial effect in disinfecting the intestine. Lactic acid (pure or as sour milk) inhibits growth of the pathogenic bacteria, allowing the healthy bifidus and coli bacteria to develop. The effect also becomes evident in the case of a severe bacterial miscolonization of the upper section of the small intestine. Germs disappear and the danger of rising bile duct infection is prevented. In diseases of the small intestine and bile duct, this diet is particularly important (preparation according to diet II A, III and IV).

Notes on Choice of Foods

Substances containing starch and sugar
Starch is present in potatoes and cereals. Various forms of preparation can be found in the recipe section. Sugar should only be used in small amounts, in the form of fruits, dried fruits and honey. White flour, industrial sugar and chocolate must be avoided.

Substances containing protein
High quality protein can be found in green leaves, whole cereals, fresh soy, nuts, milk and eggs. After tolerance has been established, milk is used for intestinal diseases in the form of types of sour milk (buttermilk, yoghurt, Bioghurt, soured milk, junket, whey). Casein is contained in quark. Cheese should only be used in small amounts and in the form of fine, mild, low fat white cheese types. Fatty, spicy, ripened types of cheese contain saturated fats, animal proteins, excessive salt and biogeneous amines produced by fermentation. They are not conducive to good health.

For a long time, the biological value of protein was calculated according to the amino-acid spectrum. These methods have not been able to stand up to more recent review. It has become clear that the combination of two or more protein types is in all cases of higher biological value than that of the protein types alone. It has been demonstrated that meat and milk proteins are not of the highest value, but can be surpassed in biological value by combinations such as potato protein with egg protein, green leaf protein with whole-grain protein, and corn protein with bean protein. Also it has been demonstrated was that pure vegetable protein combinations could easily provide the organism with the highest value protein and that the dogmatic view that animal proteins had a higher value is just not justified.

Fats
Moderate intake of fat is highly recommended. If possible, use only high-quality (not overheated) fat rich in unsaturated fatty acids and do not heat it in the kitchen. Cold pressed vegetable oils (cereal oils, sunflower oil, rapeseed oil, nut oil, sesame oil, flax seed oil) must never be heated, since they may then produce carcinogenic substances. Olive oil is recommended for hot dishes. It may be hated gently up to 170 °C, but not beyond. Vegetable margarines are hardened by physical changes to the molecules. More recent examinations indicate a detrimental metabolic effect. Fresh butter and cream should be used sparingly because of their high content of saturated fatty acids. Roasted, baked and fried dishes are not healthful.

Irritants
Irritants such as alcohol-containing drinks, coffee, black tea, chocolate, white sugar, tobacco and hot spices (e.g. pepper, hot mustard, ginger and sweet pepper) should be avoided entirely if the patient is suffering from gastrointestinal diseases, since such irritants prevent adjustment of the vagal digestion phase via the vegetative nervous system and impair digestion by irritating the mucosa. More generally they delay all regulation processes.

Hot spices should be replaced by fresh herbs. Barbecuing and roasting should be avoided because of the mucosa-irritating and roasted carcinogenic substances. Because of the contamination of the seas with chemical and radioactive waste, natural rock salt (i.e., neither iodate nor fluorinated) is safer than sea salt, unless the sea salt comes from a reliable source. People with intact kidney function should not use more than 5 g of table salt per day.

Organically biological quality
Where possible it is important to procure food grown in healthy, rich top soil that is as free from pesticides and nitrites as is feasible. This is not always possible. Nevertheless, we would like to emphasize that when following the instructions given here, important and essential protection and successful healing can be achieved, since the main relief of the gastrointestinal tract and the metabolism is achieved by dispensing with meat, fish, cheese, sugar, roasted substances, additives and irritants, and animal-based foods in general.

Diet Types

All important information on the foods making up the healing diet for digestive diseases is included in the appendix and tables.

Diet I Tea Fasting

For acute gastrointestinal catarrh, cramps and feverish digestive diseases and diarrhoea, as well as caecal colitis (if surgery can be avoided; otherwise do not eat or drink!). For strong meteorism as pre-treatment:

750–1000 g (¾ to 1 litre) tea.

Suitable teas are: chamomile (always brew briefly, should be light yellow), flaxseed, rose hip, tormentilla, marshmallow root, centaury, bitter tea, flatulence tea, blueberry, blackberry and strawberry leaf teas, unsweetened with 5–10 drops of lemon juice per glass (also see recipe section).

Bed rest, even warmth, hot abdominal compresses, Priessnitz compresses, chamomile enema with 1 litre of chamomile tea (repeat 2–3-times until the result is pure water).

Diet II Juices

A. *For Acute Diarrhoea*
(Different versions, depending on medical prescription.)

Summer catarrh, infection, sprue (coeliac disease)
After tea fasting for one day:

1 apple day
(Constipates, cleans, calms, provides nutrition of high quality fresh content.) Suitable for *all* diarrhoea types: 5–6 times per day (1 kg apples total).
Peel 1 large ripe, juicy apple, use a centrifugal juicer for the juice or grate on the Bircher grater, and then immediately eat by the spoonful. Take your time. A few drops of lemon juice prevent it from turning brown. From the second day onwards, banana beaten into a creamy consistency can be added to the grated apple. Then add more pureed food in compliance with the rules for pureed food indicated in diet III.

Or:

1 strawberry day
(Especially for sprue and chronic intestinal catarrh due to bad fat utilisation.) With a fork mash 1 kg sweet, ripe strawberries, without sugar, into a thin mash and consume during 5–6 meals. The strawberries have a particularly healing effect on coeliac disease (sprue) and severe infectious diarrhoea (paratyphus, shigelloses, rota virus infection). They have a high content of vitamins C and A, calcium, potassium and many other trace elements, at the same time a disinfecting quality and high nutritional value.

Or:

1 buttermilk day

After exclusion of milk intolerance
After one day of tea fasting, particularly suitable for summer diarrhoeas in Southern tropical climates where fruit may cause infection. Fastest change of the intestinal bacterial flora, fat-free food high in minerals. May be continued for a longer time if there is great body heat and perspiration, possibly alternating with the fresh juice diet. 1 litre *fresh* buttermilk drunk in 5–6 glasses over the course of the day. No other food except for herbal tea as described in 'fresh juices and gruel diet'.

Or:

Fresh juices and gruel diet
(For diarrhoea after apple diet.)
After a day of tea fasting and an apple day, mix juices with ⅓ rice or barley gruel or a little cream or serve in the form of pectin heads. As especially effective for diarrhoea as juice or mash are:

Fruit juices
Blueberries, grapefruit, strawberries, black currants, apples and bananas whisked and mixed with other fruit juices, and stone fruit *juices only after the diarrhoea ends.*

Vegetable juices
Carrots, beetroot, tomatoes, cabbage, celery, head lettuce.
Initially avoid:
Spinach, horseradish, cress, onion, garlic, sauerkraut.

Milk (if tolerated)
Buttermilk, much diluted almond milk, much diluted sesame milk, much diluted soy milk, mild whey, natural, lean and mild yoghurt.

Example of a day's menu
(Also see diet II, B 'Full juices'.)

When thirsty
(Patients with diarrhoea suffer badly from thirst.)
Tormentilla tea, strawberry leaf tea, blueberry tea, blackberry leaf tea, peppermint tea, chamomile tea, possibly flatulence tea. (Avoid black tea because of its content of theine and caffeine and its sleep-preventing effect; may be replaced by caffeine-free Infré tea.)

General measures for acute intestinal catarrh
Chamomile enema: use 1 litre of chamomile tea, briefly steeped (and with one soupspoon of healing earth) every 2 days.
Foo cramps: hot compresses.
Body compresses at night, after thoroughly warming the body.
Strict bed rest while there are a temperature and liquid stool.

'Kousa days'
Diet of wheat gel according to Dr. Kousa. Can be used for individual days or up to one week. Do not use for coeliac disease! Calming in case of stomach and intestinal catarrh, cleansing, slightly laxative, draining and detoxifying in case of obesity. Very mild and neutral taste but satiating. Suitable for acute gastro-intestinal catarrh, after tea fasting, apple or strawberry day, one to several days as transition to mash diet. 3–4 times daily 1 portion of wheat gel, (prepared as instructed). Served with yoghurt, fruit juice, cream, milk, raisins or oranges. If preferred slightly spiced, the wheat gel can be made more tasteful with salt-free Cenovis spice, herbs, vegetable bouillon. For recipe, see page 62.

B. For Overly Acidic Stomach, Ulcers

Juice fasting in bed
After 1 day of tea fasting (see page 52) or immediately for 2–3 days:

600–800 g fresh juices throughout the day (fruit and vegetable juices).
Prepare them of compost-fertilised (organic/biological) quality if possible.
Mixed with gruel as required.

Fruit juice types
Oranges (if tolerated), grapefruit, tangerines, grapes, berries, apples, peaches, sweet plums, melons, cherries, freshly pressed and mixed with ½ gruel (flax seed, whole wheat gel if tolerated, rice, barley), cream, pectin or agar-agar and added to the fruit juice. For severe meteorism, do not use sweet fruits.

Vegetable-juice types
Carrots, beetroots, tomatoes, lettuce, spinach, cress (by the spoonful, once tolerated), celery, fennel, horseradish, always freshly pressed and mixed with ⅓ gruel gel, agar-agar, pectin or ⅓ cream (as for fruit juices); daily cabbage juice (if possible only compost fertilised) 100 g; and potato juice 50 g. Juices may also be drunk pure or added to other juices. Flax seed gruel or whole-wheat gel: 2–5 cups, sipped throughout the day. For preparation of the gruels, see recipe part (page 62).

For stomach burn
Healing earth with chamomile tea, brewed briefly, 3–5 times 1 teaspoon per day.
Other calming medication (phytotherapy, homoeopathy, allopathy) must be chosen by the doctor. Nux vomica C 30 is often effective particularly: 6 times/day 1 drop or 4 grains.

Full juice diet
2–3 days of juice fasting in bed are followed by 2–7 days of 'full juice diet'. The following are given in addition to the fresh juices named:
almond milk,* yoghurt milk or certified raw milk (if not oversensitive, which would be recognisable from flatulence and pain), junket, sesame or soy milk, mild and fresh buttermilk, whey.**

Example of a day's menu

Morning and evening
200 g fruit juice gruel creamy mix
150 g almond milk* or soy milk; or pectin heads, 150 g fruit juice and a little cream, 150 g mild natural yoghurt.

Lunch
200 g fruit or vegetable juice mix,
140 g buttermilk or whey
or yoghurt or certified raw milk.
Cabbage juice and potato juice: 150 g flaxseed gruel every evening in case of pain at night.

For thirst
Tea types as described in diet I.
Uncarbonated mineral water (type chosen by the doctor).

General measures
Mostly bed rest, hot compresses after eating.

---

* Finely ground almonds, chewed thoroughly or prepared as milk, have a particularly healing, acid-binding and calming effect on the stomach walls. They act on the stomach like a film but without the acid-binding effect of medication.

** Whey: liquid residue from rennet cheese production, consisting of the sugars, mineral substances and vitamins of milk that are not soluble in fat. A fat-free, easily digestible, high-quality drink, predominantly alkaline in the metabolism.

After thoroughly warming up the body, apply cold body compress for the night.
Relaxation, breathing.
Chamomile enema 1 litre every 2 days.

For stomach burn
Healing earth with briefly steeped chamomile tea between the meals and in the evening 2 × 1 teaspoon.

C. For Acid-Deficient Stomach

After 1 day of tea fasting or immediately 2–3 days of full juices. Fruit and raw vegetable juices as in diet II–B, but without gruel.

Fruit juices
Grapefruit, orange, lemon diluted, all kinds of berries, sour apples, ripe stone fruit.

Vegetable juices
Spinach, horseradish, sauerkraut, sauerkraut water, sea water, lettuce, other raw vegetables.

Milk
Sour milk, yoghurt, sour buttermilk, whey (whole milk is usually badly tolerated when not soured and cause bloatedness and flatulence). Salivate well, chew slowly, and warm the food in the mouth. In rare cases a low-acid stomach will be so irritated that it will react to sour juices at first. In such cases, add ⅓ gruel to the juices, especially flax seed gruel in the juices and in sips between. This has an alleviating effect, will promote peristalsis and at the same time acts as a laxative.

Example of a day's menu

Morning
Fruit juice 200 g, yoghurt or buttermilk 150 g.

Lunch
Fruit juice 150 g, vegetable juice 150 g, yoghurt or buttermilk or sour milk 150 g.

Evening
Fruit juice or vegetable juice 200 g, yoghurt or buttermilk 150 g.

When thirsty
Acid-promoting teas such as 'bitter tea', juniper juice (by the spoonful), marshmallow-root tea, centaury tea, peppermint tea, yarrow tea, wormwood tea.
Acid-promoting vegetable bouillon with stimulating kitchen herbs, yeast spices and soy spices: 1–2 cups per day.
Mineral water, also carbonated.
Water or sea water with lemon juice added, but without sugar.

General measures
Eat slowly and salivate thoroughly. Take regular rest before meals and short naps in the afternoon. Hiking and mild gymnastics (abdominal muscles) are also beneficial.
Stomach massage by vibration, connective-tissue massage of the stomach segments, alternating hot and cold abdominal washes (i.e. affusions or hot compresses followed by cold washes). Body compresses at night after walking to warm up thoroughly. Chamomile enema every other day during the juice diet.

Diet III Pureed Food (Mash)

For stomachs with either too much or not enough acid, after stomach surgery and after intestinal catarrh, the pureed diet III follows the stage-II diet and provides a gradual transition to the solid diet. It contains all important nutritional values in a harmonious balance, so that there will be no deficiencies even if used for an extended period. The diet also permits satiation and further healing by providing adequate nutrition. This is a complete diet with refined mechanical preparation. Individual adjustment of this diet is particularly important.

This diet is suitable if the patient is hypersensitive to fat, animal protein or milk, or if he or she has a strong desire for milk casein protein.

It is also helpful where there is a tendency towards much gas formation because of vitamin C or vitamin B deficiency, sensitivity to certain fruit or vegetable types, garlic or onions, etc.

Intolerances of this kind are often overestimated and a number of foods, food groups and combinations are removed permanently and anxiously avoided because of past intolerances.

A number of mutually contradictory food theories place great importance on such rules.

However, we often see that such intolerances will slowly but surely disappear with the right approach, and that the patients will again be able to enjoy *the entire range of healthful foods that the organism requires*.

Fear must not become systematic, even though the observation of individual response to weaknesses is required, especially at the beginning.

Dietetic guidelines for pureed diet

Fresh fruit, finely grated or mashed
Apples, peaches, melons, etc. Whisked bananas, mashed. Berries, unheated and as fresh as possible. Cooked fruit must be an exception, since it cannot replace fresh fruit.

Fresh vegetables
Prepared raw in the blender or very finely chopped, mixed and served with small quantities of cream, flaxseed oil, lemon juice and almond puree (see salad dressings). Mixing and chopping must always take place right before eating (screen or blender).

Milk
All types as tolerated, pure or in mixed salads or pureed fruit, soups, Birchermuesli. Yoghurt and buttermilk are preferred to sweet whole milk.
Then soy, almond and sesame milk; whey.

Dairy products
Quark as required, mixed with herbs and acid promoters (yeast spices, soy spices or similar) either pure or mild, or with fruit juice and honey. Sunflower oil or flaxseed oil, cheeses eaten, in very small quantities: Gala, Gervais, Louis, Petit Suisse. No fat, ripe or cooked cheeses.
Sugars: fruit concentrates, naturally sweet fruit juices, small quantities of honey, stevia, no white sugar.

Cereals
Only whole cereal as gruel (Dr. Kousas whole wheat gel, whole rice, barley, oat gruel), flour (Getreidedym, Holle, etc.). Fine meal mash, well broken down, oats, barley, rice, wheat in soup form.

Potatoes
Peeled as mash and puree, not roasted.

Fat
Cold-pressed, polyunsaturated high quality plant oils, particularly sunflower, flaxseed or seed oil (must never be heated!). Olive oil contains monounsaturated fatty acids. It is suitable in combination with flaxseed oil, especially for inflammation.

A little cream may be added to the muesli or to soups if weight gain is desired. Otherwise add flaxseed oil to the muesli. Olive oil may be heated. If weight gain is desired, olive oil may be added to the soup in small amounts.
Margarines, hydrogenated and heated fats should not be used.

Drinks
All herbal teas named in diets II A, B, C, mineral water and fresh juices on demand.

Avoid
Alcohol, tobacco, coffee, white sugar, white flour, mustard, pepper, sweet pepper, curry, hot dressings, and roasted or breaded foods.
All foods should be eaten strained and well salivated.

Example of a day's menu

Morning
Birchermuesli with almond puree or yoghurt in the blender, or wheat gel or gruel soup and fruit, fruit juice with a little cream if weight gain is desired. A little crisp bread or diet rusk with quark or a little fresh butter and honey may be added to this. Herbal teas according to diet I.

Lunch
Banana and orange, whisked with a little almond milk and, if weight gain is desired, with a little cream.
2–3 raw vegetables mixed in the blender. Mashed potatoes. Mashed cooked vegetables, mineral water. Compote or fruit jelly.

Evening
Birchermuesli with almond puree or natural yoghurt and fruit juice, or junket and fruit juice.

Fresh grain cereal mash or vegetable bouillon (stirred with egg or natural), unpeeled potatoes, herbal tea.

Between meals
If thirsty drink tea, fruit juice, buttermilk.

General measures
As in diet I.

Example of a day's menu for patients with coeliac disease
(After completing juice diet II on page 52.)

Morning and evening
Birchermuesli without oat flakes through Turmix with almond milk or with certified gluten-free millet flakes
1 glass almond milk
1 whisked banana with quark
1 teaspoon linseed oil

Lunch
1 ground apple, possibly with a whisked banana
Mixed raw salad, prepared with cold-pressed flaxseed oil and lemon
Rice gruel soup (or millet or soy; never wheat, barley, spelt or rye!) or mashed potatoes or lentil puree
Arobon mash (carob flour)

Afternoon snack
Arobon mash or ground apple or whisked banana and soy flakes
Tea if thirsty (chamomile, tormentilla)

General measures
Body compress, sunlamp, calcium nutritional salts (Weleda)

Diet IV Bland Healing Diet

After completing stage-III diet: during convalescence after gastrointestinal diseases, for another 2–3 months.
For chronic slight intestinal catarrh, food hypersensitivities, sensitive stomach.
This diet corresponds largely to the Bircher-Benner regular diet, but still requires careful mechanically prepared and selected composition and the observation of particularly high quality and purity demands.
Excessive amounts of all kinds of food must be avoided.
The physiological economy in nutrition often plays a decisive role in the healing of stomach and intestine. Thorough chewing of all foods with attention to the flavour qualities restores the natural ability to choose and the feeling of satiation, so that excesses will be prevented once the patient has closely observed his sense of taste. The bland healing diet should be simple. Use of too much variety in the meal and complicated dishes, sauces/dressings, etc. should be avoided. Diet IV does not focus on care and protection, but on training the instinct and strengthening the degree of healing achieved. If a gastrointestinal disease has any purpose, it is that of experiencing such a disease with its suffering and limitations as an opportunity to get to know oneself, to take back control of oneself, and to find a desire for and pleasure in the enjoyments and activities of life that do not harm health but promote it. Therapy then becomes a fascinating experience that leads to the development of personality and maturity. Convalescence from a gastrointestinal disease is not only in diet adjustment for the long term, but also in determination of mental causes that have contributed to the occurrence of the disease. Very often the peaceful time enforced by the disease leads to new strength and, with the help of a doctor, a decisive step that makes it possible to finally overcome long-standing worry, uncertainty, accumulated anxiety or feelings of guilt.

Dietetic basics for diet IV

Simple preparation. Never use more than one type of fruit, one or two types of fresh vegetables (lettuces), or one or two vegetable dishes at once. Only in exceptional cases may you cook au gratin, with onion sautéed in butter and with a little mayonnaise. Irritants such as roasted or baked food, chocolate, coffee, tea, confectionery, alcohol and tobacco are always prohibited. Three meals per day. Small interim meals should only be eaten in exceptional cases. The food should be prepared as naturally and gently as possible. *Fruit and fresh vegetables* of all kinds and compositions should, where necessary, be chopped as finely as possible. Salads should not be prepared using strong, hot spices and herbs, but with mild, fresh herbs. The quality of fruits and vegetables is very important. Use the best available, if possible compost-fertilised bio-dynamic produce. Fruits and vegetables should not be cooked, but steamed so that their nutrients are not washed out in the cooking water, which is discarded. Salt sparingly, using high-quality rock salt or sea salt of known origin. Use vegetable broth instead of water. Cabbage types are more difficult to digest when cooked than raw. Apart from this, all fruits and vegetables should be prepared without flour-based sauces (and without onions in this diet).

Potato dishes
'Natural', mashed, puree. No roasted dishes.

Cereal dishes
Wholemeal, crisp bread, pumpernickel, diet rusk, semolina, Maizena, Mondamin, Sago and similar flours should only be used sparingly as a binder.
Corn, millet, barley, oats (whole rice) as a soup, mash or grouts.

Pastry should, if at all, be made of wholemeal and eaten no more than once a week.

Egg: should be used rarely (as an exception) and in small amounts in this bland diet.

Fat: plant oils with polyunsaturated fatty acids (must never be heated). Preferred in cold dishes (flaxseed oil, sunflower oil, safflower oil, rapeseed oil, sesame oil). A small quantity of certified cream should be used only by persons who need to gain weight. Fresh butter should only be used very sparingly, no more than 5 g/day, and only as a spread, not for cooking. Baking, roasting and frying must be avoided. Olive oil contains monounsaturated fatty acids and therefore may be slightly heated, but never above 170 °C. In salad dressings, olive oil should be combined with flaxseed oil to add the most important omega-3 oleic acids.

Milk and milk products and drinks
As in diet III.

For nutrition and scientific reasons, we recommend not eating meat or fish. Often-praised fish oils are destroyed by heating and can be replaced by the more valuable omega-3 fatty acid content of flaxseed oil. In our experience, cravings for meat will stop within 2–3 months, and often turn to aversion after the entire digestive system has been converted to a natural and harmonious diet low in irritants.

Diet V Protective Healing Diet

Expansion of the bland healing diet IV. Healthful, normal permanent diet. Prevents disease. Corresponds to stage-IV diet of our other diet books.
This diet mostly corresponds to stage-IV diet, but is more flexible and diverse.

Crisp bread, wholemeal mash, cereal meal and sprouted grains are permitted as wholemeal food. Slightly more elaborate dishes may be prepared occasionally for celebrations and diversity. This should not be done more than once a week (e.g. on Sunday). The basics of the diet should remain simple. The meals must always start with fruit and a drink. Then there should be no drinking during the meal to avoid diluting the stomach content. The share of raw fresh food (raw diet) must remain at 70 % and be enjoyed before warm foods. Alcohol, white sugar, white flour products, coffee and tobacco must be eliminated. Thus the digestive system will remain healthy, and relapses reliably avoided.

Permanent Diet for Frequent Constipation

For chronic constipation, nutritional change must be performed courageously and consistently. Laxatives must be discontinued. The lazy intestine must be given the opportunity and time to relearn its tasks. It must not be given continuous help with chemical or herbal (Senna) laxatives all the time. This would only increase its paralysis and inertia. The simplest, fastest path is to change nutrition to pure raw food for three to six weeks. Often an important change in the intestinal milieu occurs during the first week, and the peristalsis improves. It is very important to comply with regular daily schedules and get sufficient rest, alternating with abundant movement. Hiking, stimulation of the abdominal muscles and the intestine by gymnastics, alternating hot and cold showers, dry brushing and cool slapping invigorate the intestine and help it heal. It may be helpful to massage the abdomen by rubbing it clockwise in circles, ideally with a cold wet hand, as recommended by Sebastian Kneipp. This often has a surprisingly good effect. According to Kuhne, a friction hip bath leaves a pleasant freshness and invigorates the intestine and the perineum. If the first raw diet week is not enough after years of constipation, another two weeks can be added until the intestine regularly empties easily and entirely 1–3 times a day. This is usually achieved when persisting with this diet. The only additional measure must be 1–2 tablespoons of flaxseed flour (Linusit) and psyllium seeds, soaked in warm water for ½ hour, or flaxseed tea, and dried fruit, rhubarb (raw or cooked), wheat meal or bran products. Once constipation has been overcome, carefully switch from raw diet to high-quality regular diet (permanent diet IV to V). White flour, white bread, white sugar, chocolate, coffee and alcohol must now be strictly avoided at all times.

The raw food diet should be maintained for one or two days a week to be on the safe side. Do not forget careful chewing, slow eating, fresh air, gymnastics and walking.

Consequences of chronic constipation
Rectum expansion and inflammation, haemorrhoids, anal fissures, sphincter cramps.
These make healing of constipation more difficult and must be examined and treated by a doctor.

Example of a raw food day
(Permanent diet for constipation: 2–3 weeks.)

Morning
Birchermuesli of mixed fruits with almond milk or natural yoghurt and fruit, herbal tea and 1 teaspoon honey.
Sprouted wheat, nuts, dried fruit.

Lunch
Various fruit, three different types of lettuce, plenty of green leaves!
Dried fruit, nuts, sprouted grains.
Buttermilk or natural apple juice.

Evening
Same as morning, possibly replacing muesli with wheat or oat bran or adding it to the muesli.
Dried fruit, fresh fruit.

As an additive when transitioning to the regular diet: wholemeal bread with no more than 5 g butter, steamed vegetables, potatoes and wholemeal food.

The Recipes

Juices

Juices are from raw fruits and vegetables in a mechanically prepared form, used as an additional special enrichment and when coarse food (cellulose) is not permitted. Whole raw vegetables are always higher in nutritional quality and cannot be permanently replaced by juice.

For the preparation of juices, raw vegetables must be cleaned thoroughly, pressed with a hand press or an electrical centrifugal juicer, and served immediately. Any resting time reduces their value.

If a small hand press is used, fruits and vegetables must be chopped. Grate apples, pears and all bulbous vegetables finely; chop leafy vegetables and herbs finely.

Fruit Juices
Unmixed fruit juices
Orange, tangerine, grapefruit, apple, pear, grape, strawberry, blueberry, currant, cassis, raspberry, peach, apricot, plum, mango, Japanese persimmon (kaki), kiwi.

Mixed fruit juices
(Citrus fruits only if there is no oversensitivity to them.)
Orange, tangerine, grapefruit, Japanese persimmon (kaki) or berry juice with apple juice (or berry juice with peach), apricot or plum juice (or mashed bananas) with orange, berry, peach, mango or apricot juice.

Additions to taste or as needed: lemon juice, honey, maple syrup, fruit concentrate, cream, yoghurt, almond milk, flaxseed, rice or barley gruel.

Vegetable Juices
When fresh they have a high mineral and vitamin content. Each juice has its own special value.

Unmixed vegetable juices
Tomato, carrot, beetroot, radish, cabbage, celery, and all leaf, bulb and root vegetables; stinging nettle, sorrel and dandelion juice for springtime blood-cleansing treatment.

Mixed vegetable juices
Carrot, tomato, and spinach in equal proportions (very good flavour)
tomato and carrot.
Tomato and spinach.

Other mixes (and cocktails) can be combined to taste.

For variety, add sorrel, stinging nettle, chives, parsley, onions, tender celery leaves or roots, and other herbs.

Additions per glass (1½–2 dl): 1 teaspoon cream, almond puree or buttermilk, a little lemon juice, fruit concentrate (optional, small quantity). Flaxseed (optional), rice or barley gruel. Other leafy vegetables or lettuces may be used, such as white cabbage, endives, field, lamb's lettuce, lettuce, dandelion.

Potato juice:
Prepare scrubbed, peeled (optional) potatoes (no unripe, green or sprouted ones) like carrot juice. Not tasty, but relieves

cramps and is particularly effective for heartburn and for stomach and duodenal ulcers.

Gruel to Accompany Juices
The gruel is added to raw juices at a proportion of 1:3. It neutralises the sharpness of the fruit or vegetable flavour. The daily ration can be prepared once a day and kept in a thermos bottle.

Rice or barley gruel:
Stir 1 heaped teaspoon rice or barley wholemeal flour with 2 dl cold water and boil for 5 min., stirring constantly. Let cool.

Linseed gruel:
Rinse 1 tablespoon flaxseeds, boil in 2 dl water for 10 min., strain and let cool.

Wheat Gel (Dr. Kousa)*
50 g dry weight served in 4–5 portions per day.
Preparation as indicated on the packaging.

Healthful Teas

Use whole leaves for teas if possible, since essential oils are lost when the leaves are chopped more finely (sachet form). Bitter and flatulence teas should be drunk unsweetened, while other teas may be enhanced with honey and/or lemon juice.

Bitter tea
Wormwood
Centaurium
Cnicus

Mix in equal parts, boil briefly and steep for 5 min.
To stimulate the appetite, drink 2–3 tablespoons ½ hour before meals
(mildly cholagogic); aids in digestion.
Sensitive persons should use only centaurium (prepared like camomile tea).

Wormwood tea
Boil briefly and steep for 5 min.
Strong bitter tea, strongly cholagogic, stimulates gastric juices.
Drink in sips throughout the day.

Flatulence tea
Caraway
Fennel
Aniseed
Mix in equal parts, boil briefly and steep for 20 min.
Drink 1 cup after meals to prevent flatulence.

Chamomile tea
Boil briefly.
For stomach pain.
Cleansing and calming effect on the gastrointestinal tract.
For enemas and rinsing.

Peppermint tea
Boil briefly.
Calming, cholagogic, stimulates the small intestine.

Vervain tea
Boil briefly.
Calming, mucous reducing, cholagogic; very popular tea in France, drunk in the afternoon and evening.

Lemon balm tea
Boil briefly.
Very calming, good before bedtime.

Orange blossom tea
Boil 2–3 blossoms for 2–3 min., let steep and strain. Sweeten with honey.
Calming; drink at bedtime.

Flaxseed tea
Boil 1 tablespoon flaxseeds in ½ l water for 7–10 min. and let steep.
Mucous reducing, mildly laxative, calms the stomach.

---

* See page 98.

Bearberry leaf tea
Briefly boil 1½ tablespoons bearberry leaves in 5 dl water for 5 min., steep for 10 min. and strain.
For bladder infections.

Lavender tea
Briefly boil 1 teaspoon lavender leaves, steep briefly.
Calming, harmonising, anti-inflammatory: for sleeplessness.

Rosehip tea
Soak 2–3 tablespoons rosehip seeds and peels in 1½ l water for 12 hours, boil gently for ½–¾ hours and strain. The next day, the boiled rosehips can be boiled again with fresh ones.
Slightly cholagogic and diuretic, refreshing and stimulating.

Yarrow tea
(Prepared like chamomile tea.) Stimulates the stomach, relieves cramps, heals inflammation, styptic.

Strawberry leaf tea
(Prepared like peppermint tea.)
Slightly constipating.

Marshmallow root tea
1 tablespoon in ¼ l water, cook for 5 min, steep for 10 min, strain. Gastrointestinal cleaning and calming.

Tormentill tea
(Prepared like marshmallow root tea.)
Cleans the intestines, slightly constipating.

Blueberry tea
1 tablespoon dried blueberries, soak for 12 hours and cook for 5 minutes. Strain.
Relieves constipation, calming.

Muesli

All recipes are for 1 person.

The apple muesli
In our long experience, the original apple muesli as invented by Dr Bircher and used successfully thousands of times with his patients has remained the best food for the regime.

Sweet-tart juicy apples with white flesh are best for the muesli (e.g. Klar, Gravenstein, Sauergrauech, Menznauer Jäger, Jonathan, Ontario, Rubinette, Glockenäpfel, Braeburn, Champagner-Reinetten, Cox's Orange).

The flavour of drier apple types with a weaker taste can be enriched with a pinch of the freshly ground peel of untreated oranges or lemons, or with orange juice, a little rosehip paste or freshly grated ginger.

Sugar, honey, nuts and almonds must only be used if permitted by the doctor, and never during an acute stage of a gastrointestinal disease.

Apple muesli with yoghurt, sour milk or buttermilk
1 tablespoon oat flakes
3 tablespoon water
2 tablespoon Bifidus yoghurt, Bifidus sour milk or buttermilk
1 teaspoon honey
200 g apples
1 tablespoon hazelnuts or almonds, grated

Soak the oat flakes for 12 hours (overnight if for breakfast). Mix the oat flakes, yoghurt (or sour milk) and honey into a smooth sauce. Remove stems and calyxes from the washed apples and grate the apples with the Bircher grater into the sauce. Stir several times to keep the muesli pleasantly white. Spread the nuts on it and serve at once. Never let it rest.

Versions: Replace oat flakes with wheat, rice, barley, rye, semolina, buckwheat or soy flakes, optionally mixed with yeast flakes (enriching with vitamin B).

Another version: Mix 1 teaspoon soaked oat flakes with 1 teaspoon cereal grains (whole, chopped or mixed). Soak in water for 24 hrs. then put through a sieve and rinse with cold water.

Muesli with almond or sesame puree
(If animal protein is forbidden in allergies.)
1 tablespoon oat flakes
3 tablespoons water
½ tablespoon lemon juice
1 tablespoon almond or sesame puree
1 tablespoon honey
3 tablespoons water
200 g apples
1 tablespoon hazelnuts or almonds, grated

Soak oat flakes for 12 hours. Stir in lemon juice, puree, honey and water with a whisk to produce a creamy consistency, add the oat flakes and apples (prepared like basic recipe). Spread the nuts on top and serve at once.

Apple muesli with cream
(Specially enriched recipe if weight gain is desired.)
1 teaspoon (8 g) fine oat flakes
3 tablespoons water
½ teaspoon lemon juice
3–4 tablespoons cream
1 tablespoon honey
200 g apples
1 tablespoon hazelnuts or almonds, ground

Prepared like basic recipe.

Muesli with berries or stone fruit
(Particularly rich in vitamin C.)
Prepare an almond puree or sesame puree or yoghurt sauce. Add
150–200 g strawberries or raspberries, blueberries, currants or blackberries, and mash slightly with a fork.
Or
150–200 g plums, peaches or apricots, pitted and passed through the chopper or cut finely with a knife.

Muesli with various fruits
The following combinations are very tasty:

strawberries and raspberries
strawberries, raspberries and currants
strawberries and apples
blackberries and apples
apples with finely cut orange and tangerine wedges
apples and bananas
apples and peaches
sauce: almond or sesame puree sauce, or yoghurt sauce
Use only fresh fruits, never use canned fruits (fruit salad, etc.).

Muesli with dried fruits
If you have no fresh fruits to hand, you can also make the muesli with dried fruits (apples, apricots, plums, pears). One hundred grams of dried fruits are washed, soaked in cold water for 12 hours and ground through the chopper. Mix with almond or sesame puree sauce or yoghurt sauce. For dried fruits, always look for good quality without preservatives or bleach; otherwise, gastrointestinal problems may occur.

Muesli with condensed milk
If you do not have almond or sesame puree or fresh yoghurt to hand, you can make the muesli with condensed milk

according to the original recipe.
Disadvantage: condensed milk often contains added sugar.

Sprouted cereal grains
These are particularly high in the vitamin E and B group, and generally have a strengthening effect.
1st day, evening: wash the grains in a screen under running water and put them in a bowl. Cover with water and keep at room temperature, close to the oven.
2nd day, morning: rinse the grains and spread to dry on a flat plate at room temperature, close to the oven.
The same evening, put them back in the bowl and cover with water. Keep at room temperature, close to the oven.
3rd day, morning: rinse the grains and spread to dry on the plate.
Evening: put the grains back in the bowl and cover with water. Keep at room temperature, close to the oven.
On the 4th day, the grains should have developed sprouts of 1–2 cm and are ready to eat.

The preparation of sprouted cereal grains is easier in the practical sprouting devices that are available in different sizes.

Sprouted cereal grains are suitable for preparing muesli, and also go well with salads and raw vegetables.

Linomel muesli according to Dr. Johanna Budwig
1 teaspoon honey
2 tablespoons milk, gently warmed
1–2 tablespoons flaxseed oil
50–100 g low fat quark
2–3 teaspoons Linomel (flaxseed/honey granulate, available from health-food stores)
150–200 g fresh seasonal fruits
1 tablespoon sunflower seeds or ground almonds or hazelnuts

Put 2–3 tablespoons of Linomel into a small dish, add the chopped fruits (if desired, enriched with softened raisins, sultanas or raisins).
Mix honey, milk and linseed oil with a mixer or whisk, gradually add the quark and stir the mixture into a smooth, thick cream.
Pour over the fruits and spread the sunflower seeds or grated nuts on top.

Raw vegetables and salads

Observe three considerations when preparing raw vegetables and salads:

1. Freshness and quality
For the gastrointestinal diet as well as for any other diet and for everyday nutrition, use only sun-ripened, organically grown vegetables and lettuces. They are not only optimal for health but also have the best taste. Today the offer from organically run businesses is very large, and organically grown vegetables are available even in supermarkets. Of course, it is even more beneficial to use vegetables and lettuces from your own garden. Herbs and tomatoes can be grown even on a balcony. Choose young, tender leafy lettuces and root vegetables, not blanched, without any wilted leaves or rotting stalks. For a healing regime it is particularly important to use only entirely fresh and high quality plants.
Prepare raw vegetables just before eating them and mix them with the dressing immediately. Letting them stand will markedly reduce the vitamin content of the chopped vegetables and lettuces.

2. Cleanliness
Vegetables grown organically without manure fertilisation contain no worm

eggs. Nevertheless, all fresh plants must be cleaned thoroughly and carefully. Observe that water-soluble substances such as vitamin C, vitamins of the B-group and minerals are leached out in water.

3. Harmonious composition

Every salad dish should contain all three types of vegetable: root, fruit and leaf. Green leafy lettuce in particular is always part of a healing regime. A variety of dressings can be used to enhance the various ingredients of the raw food.
A beautifully assembled salad in pleasing colours is agreeable to the eye and the palate and stimulates the appetite.
Small garnishes of herbs, radishes, young carrots or olives make the raw vegetable dish even more colourful and festive. The three types of vegetable should not be exceeded per meal for everyday use. Too much variety may impair digestion.

Cleaning leafy vegetables

For head lettuce, endives, romaine lettuce, iceberg lettuce and similar green leaf lettuces, cabbage and red cabbage, separate the leaves and clean them individually and carefully under running water. Rinse several times and spin dry thoroughly.
Small leaved salads such as lamb's lettuce and cut lettuce, spinach, dandelion, cress, rocket, radicchio and Brussels sprouts should be rinsed repeatedly in small portions. Any hard stalks should be removed. Halve chicory and radicchio remove outer leaves and rinse well.

Cleaning root vegetables

Celery, carrots, horseradish, radish, beetroot, kohlrabi, black salsify: clean with a brush under running water, peel and immediately grate or slice into the finished sauce. Mix well to preserve the vegetables' fresh colour.

Cleaning vegetable fruits

Wash tomatoes and cut them into wedges or slices. Peel cucumbers and cut them small or grate them. Organically grown young cucumbers do not need to be peeled.
Use only young, tender unpeeled courgettes for salads, wash them thoroughly and slice or julienne them.
Green and yellow sweet pepper is less hot than the red variety. Wash, halve, remove seeds and cut small. Unfortunately, today almost all sweet peppers come from hydroponic production.
Separate cauliflower and broccoli into florets and clean thoroughly under running water.
Wash stalk celery, peel it, and cut away hard parts.
Halve leeks and fennel, prepare and wash under the tap set to shower.

Salad dressings

Use the various dressings as prescribed by a doctor.

Oil dressing

1 tablespoon oil (rapeseed, sunflower or olive oil from first cold pressing, thistle oil, walnut oil)
1 teaspoon lemon juice or organic fruit vinegar
optional garlic, pressed
1 teaspoon fresh herbs (or 1 knife tip dried herbs)

Mix all ingredients and whisk the dressing until creamy. The dressing is also very tasty with a splash of soy sauce or Kelpamare.
This classic salad dressing is suited to all green salads (head lettuce, romaine lettuce, cress, etc.) and fruit salads (tomatoes, cucumbers etc.).

Quark dressing
1 tablespoon lean quark
3 tablespoons buttermilk
½ teaspoon lemon juice
fresh, finely chopped herbs

Whisk all ingredients thoroughly.
This dressing goes particularly well with root vegetables (carrots, celery root (celeriac), radishes etc.)

Yoghurt dressing
(For the low-fat diet.)
2–3 tablespoons yoghurt
a few drops of lemon juice
onion, grated
garlic, pressed
1 teaspoon fresh herbs (or 1 knife tip dried herbs)

Whisk all ingredients thoroughly.
A refreshing dressing with cress or spinach, with fruit salads (tomatoes, cucumbers) and with root vegetables (kohlrabi, horseradish, radishes).

Cream dressing
2 tablespoons sour cream
1 teaspoon lean quark
1 teaspoon lemon juice
very little pepper
1 teaspoon fresh herbs (or 1 knife tip dried herbs)

Whisk all ingredients thoroughly.
This dressing suits almost all root and fruit salads. For variety you may replace lemon juice with orange juice, to give the raw food a new flavour. With celery, beetroot and chicory salad, you can add a little freshly grated horseradish to this sauce for a very stimulating taste.

Almond or sesame puree dressing
(Diet without animal protein.)
1 tablespoon almond or sesame puree
3 tablespoons water
1 teaspoon lemon juice
garlic, pressed
1 teaspoon fresh herbs (or knife tip dried herbs)

Slowly stir sesame or almond puree with water until smooth, then add the other ingredients.
This tasty dressing goes very well with root vegetables.

Classic mayonnaise recipe
For 4 persons:
1 egg yolk
1 tablespoon lemon juice
2 dl oil
onions, herbs, a little Kelpamare

Mix the yolk well with a few drops of lemon juice. Add the oil drop by drop, stirring evenly with the whisk. If the mayonnaise grows too thick, dilute with lemon juice. Season to taste.

For 1 portion:
1 tablespoon mayonnaise
1 teaspoon lemon juice
1 teaspoon fresh (or 1 knife tip dried herbs)

Mix all ingredients well.

Mayonnaise with wholegrain soy flour instead of egg
(Recipe for vegan nutrition and prohibition of animal protein.)
For 6–8 portions:
2 tablespoons soy wholegrain flour
6 tablespoons water
2 dl oil

Mix soy wholegrain flour and water until smooth. Slowly add oil while constantly stirring with the whisk.
The mayonnaise can be kept in the fridge for a few days.

For 1 portion:
1 tablespoon mayonnaise
1 teaspoon lemon juice
a touch of mustard (optional)

1 teaspoon fresh herbs (or knife tip dried herbs)

Mix all ingredients well.
Mayonnaise is a popular dressing for many fruit salads and root vegetables.

Raw vegetables, mixed
chicory with tomato dice – oil dressing or mayonnaise
sweet peppers and fennel – oil dressing
fennel, chicory and tomato dice – mayonnaise
fennel and carrots – cream dressing
cauliflower and carrots – cream dressing
tomatoes and peppers – oil dressing or mayonnaise

Tomatoes, raw, stuffed
with cucumbers – oil dressing or mayonnaise
with celery – cream dressing
with cauliflower – cream dressing

Sauerkraut salad
Sauerkraut is a particularly valuable raw vegetable, especially in winter. It is more easily digestible raw than cooked and has a gallbladder-purging and disinfecting effect. Use the low salt organic sauerkraut if possible. An addition of finely cut raw sauerkraut can considerably improve the taste and digestibility of steamed sauerkraut. For a salad, the sauerkraut is loosely separated, chopped and mixed with a few caraway seeds (or ground caraway), 3–4 chopped juniper berries, sliced onion, a julienned apple or a diced small fresh pineapple. Choose oil dressing as a dressing. This salad goes well with corn salad and a raw, root vegetables.

Mixed – pureed raw vegetables
If the doctor prescribes 'pureed diet', certain raw vegetables may be mixed with the dressing in the blender. This is the transition from juice to normal raw vegetable food.

Examples:
1 tomato 70 g, 1 handful spinach 30 g, 1 small carrot 70 g, one knife tip marjoram, with oil dressing
1 tomato 70 g, 1 handful head lettuce 20 g, 1 small piece of celery root (celeriac) 20 g, with cream dressing (with lovage)
beetroots 30 g, zucchini 40 g, head lettuce 20 g, with cream dressing (with dill)
celery 40 g, carrots 40 g, spinach 20 g, almond puree dressing (with rosemary)

Suggestions for dressings to go with the salads and raw vegetables

head lettuce	uncut	oil dressing	chives, onion
cut lettuce	uncut	oil dressing	chives, onion
endives/chicory	cut in strips of 1 cm	oil dressing	onion, parsley
lamb's lettuce	uncut	oil dressing	onion, parsley
cress	uncut	yoghurt dressing	chives
spinach	cut strips of ½ cm	yoghurt dressing	peppermint
cabbage lettuces: white cabbage, sauerkraut, Brussels sprouts, savoy cabbage	slice, cut into thin pieces	oil dressing or nut dressing	lovage, savory, thyme, caraway
tomatoes	slice or dice	oil dressing or yoghurt dressing	basil, thyme, oregano
cucumbers	slice	oil dressing	dill
fennel	finely cut with knife	cream dressing or oil dressing	dill, chives, parsley
sweet peppers	cut into fine strips	oil dressing or mayonnaise	chives
radish	slice or grate	quark dressing	chives, parsley
small radish	slice or cut finely	yoghurt dressing	chives, parsley
stalk celery	cut finely	oil dressing or almond-puree dressing	chives, thyme
courgettes	grate coarsely or slice	oil dressing or almond-puree dressing	dill, borage, basil
beets	grate finely	yoghurt or orange dressing	chives, lovage
Celery (celeriac)	grate finely	nut dressing	ginger
beetroot	grate finely	cream dressing	horseradish
cauliflower, broccoli	cut off florets, grate stems	garlic dressing	chives
chicory/endives	cut in strips of 1 cm	cream sauce	tarragon, parsley
Jerusalem artichoke	grate	mayonnaise	marjoram, thyme
kohlrabi	slice or grate	yoghurt dressing or nut dressing	thyme, lovage
red cabbage	slice or cut finely	almond-puree dressing	some grated apple, caraway, lovage

Chives, parsley and onions may be added in moderation to any raw vegetable, according to taste.

Milk Types

Almond milk
This food provides vegetable protein and oil and is rich in valuable unsaturated plant oils.
Stimulates mucous production and soothes.

1 tablespoon almond puree
1½ teaspoons honey
1½ dl water and ½ dl fruit juice (causes slight thickening)

Mix almond puree and honey with the whisk and add water drop by drop. Add fruit juice last.

Almond milk of fresh almonds
Particularly easy to digest

1½ tablespoons almonds, peeled (no bitter ones)
1 teaspoon honey
1½ dl water

Mix almonds, honey and water in the mixer. Strain if necessary.

Pine nut milk
Very rich in easily digestible vegetable oils and protein that protects the metabolism.

1½ tablespoons pine nuts, washed
1 teaspoon honey
1½ dl water

Prepare like almond milk.

Sesame milk
2 dl water (cold or warm)
1 level tablespoon sesame puree
1 teaspoon lemon juice
1 teaspoon honey

Mix sesame puree and honey with the whisk and add the water drop by drop. Add the lemon juice.

Sesame cream
Like sesame milk, but with less water added. Replaces cream in cooked dishes and desserts.

Sesame frappé (milkshake)
Like sesame milk or sesame cream, with addition of fruit juice, apple juice, fruit concentrates.

Soy milk
1 cup soy beans
7 cups water
1 tablespoon fruit sugar
water

Wash and dry soy beans and grind them in an almond mill. Soak for 2 hours, then boil for 20 min. in the water used for soaking, stirring constantly. Strain. Add water until the viscosity of cow's milk is reached. Add fructose and let cool. Soy milk is sold in tetra packs in health-food stores.

Butter, vegetable fats and oils – gentle cooking and steaming/sautéing

The Bircher cuisine uses only cold-pressed oils, almond and other nut purees for raw food. Cooked food may also be prepared using small amounts of fresh butter and olive oil. Vegetable oils generally should not be heated, since heating may turn the highly unsaturated fatty acids into harmful free radicals.

Fresh butter
To enhance dishes.

Vegetable margarine, food fats or olive oil and butter
Margarine results from hydrogenation of vegetable oils in the presence of catalysts. The catalysts emit traces of aluminium and nickel. If palm fat is used, carcinogenic glycidol fatty acid esters result. Epidemiological studies confirm that high

margarine consumption will promote cancer, in contrast to olive oil. Margarines also contain trans-fatty acid esters, which have a detrimental influence on the cholesterol metabolism. Where possible, cooking should be low in fat. A little olive oil should be used to enrich the meal (never heat above 140 °C). Use butter sparingly.

Nut spread and almond puree
These fats have a very fine, nutty flavour. They can be used variously as bland food or to replace fresh butter or vegetable margarine with vegetables, potatoes, rice, and pasta.

Cold-pressed sunflower oil, corn seed oil, thistle oil, cold-pressed olive oil
Organic and carefully treated, rich in highly unsaturated fatty acids, these fats are more easily digestible for most people than butter. However, as mentioned, the vegetable oils should not be heated, because heating may produce harmful free radicals. Flaxseed oil has a very distinctive flavour and, mixed with a little lemon juice, flaxseed oil will only go well with certain raw vegetables and the Linomel muesli (see recipe page 65). As treatment, however, it is highly recommended: 2 × 2 tablespoons per day; do not leave the oil exposed to air, but keep it tightly closed in the refrigerator. The addition of lemon juice protects against oxidation.

Gentle cooking and steaming/sautéing

Today hardly any housewife or working woman will want to do without her pressure cooker. This appliance is time-saving and far more healthful than other methods. Who would want to forgo these advantages?

The pressure cooker works especially well for soups and is useful for almost every other recipe. The cooking time is only ⅓ to ¼ of the normal cooking time. Many vegetable and potato recipes also can be steamed gently and very quickly in the pressure cooker, resulting in dishes that retain their colour, aroma, vitamins and nutrients. If you like your vegetables firmer (al dente), the cooking time of vegetables (except potatoes) can be reduced to taste, even with conventional steaming.

For cereal dishes, we recommend using the steamer for grains with long cooking times (e.g. coarse corn) but not for pasta products.

Soups

The recipes are for 1 person.

The following soup and vegetable recipes use a lot of vegetable broth. In a small household, it is inconvenient to make fresh vegetable broth every day. Instead, you may use ordinary water and salt-free vegetable bouillon cubes or pastes (also salt free). Cream enriches soups and vegetables, but milk can usually be used instead.

In case of wheat allergy, the wholegrain flour in the recipes should be replaced by rice, millet or oat flour.

Vegetable broth
Unlike other recipes in this book, this recipe is for 4 persons

1 tablespoon olive oil
1 onion
2 carrots
1 small stalk of celery (150 g)
cabbage, Swiss chard leaves
1 leek stalk
3–4 l water
½ bay leaf
1 pinch sea salt
lovage, basil or other herbs, dried or preferably fresh

Half the onion, keeping the brown peel, and brown the cut area in the hot olive oil until golden yellow. Chop the vegetables, add them and cook for at least 15 min. covered at low heat. Add water and cook for 2 hours at low heat. Season to taste.

Vegetable bouillon
3 dl vegetable broth
Kelpamare
10 g nut spread or olive oil
parsley, chives, freshly chopped herbs

Prepare the vegetable broth according to the above recipe and add to nut spread, olive oil and herbs. Add a little Kelpamare (optional).

Semolina dumplings
10 g butter
1 ½ teaspoons fine semolina
½–1 egg
1 pinch salt
marjoram, nutmeg
6 dl vegetable broth

Cream the butter until foamy. Mix the semolina and egg thoroughly with the butter. Add salt and spices and let the mix rest for ½ hour. Use a teaspoon to shape the dumplings. Place them in the boiling vegetable bouillon and let steep for 15 to 20 minutes.

Rice soup, clear
½ tablespoon olive oil
a little chopped onion
1 small carrot
a little celery and leek
1 tablespoon rice
1 pinch of salt
6 dl vegetable broth
chives

Sauté onion with finely cut vegetables and rice together. Add hot vegetable broth and cook for 15–20 minutes. Prepare with finely cut chives and olive oil.

Rice soup, thickened
½ tablespoon olive oil
a little celery and leek
1 small carrot
1 tablespoon rice
½ tablespoon wholegrain flour
6 dl vegetable broth or water
lovage, parsley, basil, marjoram
a little soya sauce (optional)
½ tablespoon cream or sesame cream (see recipe page 70)
chives

Sauté the chopped vegetables in olive oil. Sprinkle with wholegrain flour, pour on vegetable broth and cook for 30 minutes. Season with soya sauce and herbs. Place cream and finely cut chives in the soup bowl and serve the soup over them.

Herbal soup
1 tablespoon wholegrain flour
1 dl milk or water
5 dl vegetable broth
½ tablespoon cream
5 g butter, olive oil or nut spread (optional)
1 egg yolk
lovage, basil, tarragon, marjoram, chives, nutmeg or caraway (optional)

Stir wholegrain flour into cold milk or cold water and add to the boiling vegetable broth. Cook for 15 minutes. Season with the herbs. Add cream (or optional olive oil, nut spread or egg yolk) into the soup bowl, add the soup and whisk.

Oat cream soup
½ tablespoon olive oil
2 tablespoons fine or coarse oat flakes
6 dl vegetable broth
a little celery
½ tablespoon cream or sesame cream (see recipe page 70)
Optional: miso, chives, nutmeg or caraway

Briefly sauté oat flakes with or without olive oil. Add vegetable broth and celery.

Slightly cook oat flakes for 10 minutes, (coarse ones for at least 20 minutes). Season to taste. Place cream or sesame cream and chives in the soup bowl and add the pureed soup.

Oat groats soup
½ tablespoon olive oil
2 tablespoons oat groats
a little chopped onion
7 dl water or vegetable broth
1 dl milk
a little diced celery
1 pinch sea salt or some miso
1 tablespoon cream (optional)
chives, parsley, marjoram or borage

Sauté onion and groats with or without olive oil. Add vegetable broth, milk and celery and cook for 45–60 minutes. Season to taste with sea salt or miso. Place cream and herbs in the soup bowl and add the soup.

Semolina soup
1 tablespoon semolina
5 dl vegetable broth

½ tablespoon cream or sesame cream (see recipe page 70)
1 egg yolk or
5 g fresh butter or olive oil
or nut spread
1 pinch sea salt or Kelpamare
caraway, nutmeg (optional)
lovage, basil, marjoram, parsley, chives

Stir semolina into the boiling vegetable broth, add Kelpamare and caraway, and simmer for ½ hour. Season to taste with herbs. Place cream and egg yolk or olive oil or nut spread in the soup bowl and add the soup.

Tomato soup
½ tablespoon olive oil
a little onion, celery and leek
1 small carrot
1 garlic clove
1 tomato
1 tablespoon wholegrain flour
6 dl vegetable broth
1 pinch sea salt
a little tomato puree (optional)
1 pinch fruit sugar (or Succanat)
rosemary, oregano
5 g butter, olive oil or nut spread
½ tablespoon cream or sesame cream (see recipe page 70)
chives

Sauté vegetables cut small with or without olive oil, then add the tomato. Sprinkle with wholegrain flour and pour the vegetable broth into the mixture. Cook for ½ hour then strain. Add spices and tomato puree (optional). Place olive oil (or nut spread) and cream in the soup bowl and add the finished soup. Sprinkle with finely cut chives. If desired, add 1 tablespoon rice to the soup or sprinkle with fat-free toasted bread cubes.

Summer tomato soup
4 summer tomatoes
1 pinch fruit sugar (or Succanat)
1 pinch sea salt
1 tablespoon cream

Dice the tomatoes, cook briefly, season and strain. Add cream and serve the soup lukewarm or cold.

Vegetable soups (carrots, spinach, broccoli, cauliflower)
½ tablespoon olive oil
a little chopped onion
1½ tablespoons wholegrain flour
1 pinch sea salt
5 dl vegetable broth
1 dl milk
1 tablespoon cream or sesame cream (see recipe page 70)
Vegetables: 1 diced carrot or 1 small cup of spinach, pureed or finely chopped, broccoli or cauliflower finely chopped (cook some of the flowers separately and set them aside).

Sauté onion and carrots or broccoli or cauliflower with or without olive oil. Sprinkle with wholegrain flour and sauté them together briefly. Pour in vegetable broth and milk and cook for 20–40 minutes. For the spinach soup, add the spinach last and remove from heat. Pour the soup over the cream in the soup bowl. For the broccoli or cauliflower soup, add flowers previously set aside.

Seasoning: For carrot soup, use celery leaves or lovage, rosemary or marjoram, 1 teaspoon caraway.
For spinach soup, use some peppermint leaves, parsley, chives, 1 pinch of nutmeg.
For broccoli or cauliflower soup, use a little basil, parsley, chives, tarragon.

Chervil soup

½ tablespoon olive oil
a little onion
1 medium-sized potato, chopped in cubes
½ tablespoon wholegrain flour
5 dl vegetable broth
1 pinch sea salt
1 tablespoon chervil, chopped
1 tablespoon cream

Sauté the onion slightly with or without olive oil. Add potato, sprinkle with wholegrain flour and add vegetable broth and salt. Cook for ½ hour and strain. Put chervil and cream in the soup bowl and add the soup.

Potato soup

½ leek, cut into thin strips
½ carrot, sliced
½ tablespoon wholegrain flour
5 dl vegetable broth
1 medium-sized potato, diced
1 pinch sea salt or a little miso
basil, marjoram
1 tablespoon cream

Sauté the leek and carrot in a little vegetable broth. Sprinkle with wholegrain flour and add the vegetable broth. Add potato and cook until soft. Season. Put basil, marjoram and optional cream in the soup bowl and add the finished soup.

Minestrone

½ tablespoon olive oil
2 tablespoon leek
a little onion, finely chopped
a few celery leaves
½ plateful beet greens
7 dl water or vegetable broth
1 tablespoon lovage or thyme
½ garlic clove, pressed
basil, parsley, chives
1 pinch sea salt
15 g pasta or rice
5 g butter or olive oil or nut spread

Finely chop onion, leek, celery leaves and beet greens and sauté them slowly. Add vegetable broth, season and cook for ½ hour. Add pasta or rice and cook another 15–20 minutes. To enrich, add cream or nut spread or olive oil.

Vegetables

Spinach, chopped
(Do not use if suffering from diarrhoea.)
(Stage I–IV diet.)
¼ l vegetable broth
200 g spinach (remove thick stems)
¼ garlic clove, pressed
1 pinch sea salt
peppermint leaves, sage
1 cup raw spinach
optional some olive oil

Briefly cook spinach in the vegetable broth and drain, then finely cut, chop or blend. Return spinach to the pan and heat. Add garlic, salt and herbs.
Chop or blend the raw spinach and add to the cooked spinach (with a little fresh butter or olive oil) before serving.

Spinach, whole leaves (and branches)
(Do not use if suffering from diarrhoea.)
(Only on stage-V diet.)
300 g spinach (remove thick stems, briefly boil the coarser winter spinach if required)
1 tablespoon pine nuts
1 tablespoon raisins (optional)
1 pinch sea salt
peppermint leaves, sage, parsley
optional: olive oil

Steam spinach uncovered over low heat with very little water. Add pine nuts, spices and optional raisins and briefly continue cooking. Add melted butter or vegetable margarine if desired.

Lettuce
1 romaine lettuce
1 l water
a little chopped onion
½ tablespoon olive oil
1 dl vegetable broth
1 pinch sea salt

Halve the romaine lettuce, boil until semi-soft then drain. Reassemble the lettuce and place in an oven-proof mould. Lightly sauté the onion in olive oil and place it over the lettuce. Add vegetable broth and a pinch of sea salt and cook in the oven for 30–40 min.

Endives (chicory)
1 large endive head

Prepare just like romaine lettuce.

Sautéed chicory (endive)
2 heads chicory
½ tablespoon olive oil
3 tablespoons vegetable broth
1 pinch sea salt
marjoram, thyme
a little butter or olive oil or nut spread

Halve the chicory (endive) and layer the leaves in the pan. Add heated olive oil and vegetable broth to the chicory (endive), season and cook covered over low heat for ½ hour. At the end, spread melted butter or olive oil or nut spread on the prepared vegetables.

Chard (Swiss chard) with béchamel sauce
(Do not use if suffering from meteorism.)
(Only on stage-V diet.)
3 chards
½ tablespoon olive oil
½ dl vegetable broth
a little lemon juice or 1 tablespoon almond puree
1 pinch sea salt
tarragon, parsley and chives
béchamel sauce (see recipe page 87)

Cut the chard leaves into pieces of 3 cm., sauté in olive oil. Add vegetable broth and lemon juice or almond puree and cook covered over low heat for ½ to ¾ hour until soft. Season and mix the fresh vegetables with béchamel sauce.

Celery stalks
3–4 stalks celery
½ onion, chopped
a little apple, finely chopped
1 dl vegetable broth
1 teaspoon almond puree
1 pinch sea salt or
a little soya
celery greens

Cut the celery stalk into pieces 8 cm long and place in a pan. Briefly sauté the onion and apple without fat and spread on the celery. Add vegetable broth and almond puree and cook over low heat for ½ to ¾ hour until soft. Season.

Baked fennel with cream cheese
1 large or 2 small fennel plants
1 pinch sea salt
pepper
several drops of lemon juice
1 cream cheese

Quarter the fennel and steam it until semi-soft. Pull apart the individual layers of the fennel bulb and place them in an oven-proof mould. Drizzle with lemon juice, then salt and pepper. Stir the cream cheese with 2 tablespoons of fennel stock and spread on the vegetables. Bake in a hot oven.

Vegetable curry
1 tablespoon sun flower oil
1 spring onion
200 g vegetables (e.g. leeks, carrots, courgettes, asparagus)
½ teaspoon wholegrain flour
1 knife tip (to taste) curry powder
½ teaspoon vegetable broth
½ orange
1 teaspoon sultanas
1 pinch whole-cane sugar (or Succanat)
1 pinch sea salt, pepper

Cut the spring onion into fine rings and cook in slightly heated oil. Sprinkle flour and curry powder and add the vegetable broth. Add the cut small vegetables and cook covered for approx. 15 minutes. Set aside two or three wedges of the orange, squeeze the rest and place the sultanas in the juice. When the vegetables are soft, add the sultanas and orange juice, heat the mixture and season with sugar, salt and pepper. Serve and spread the orange wedges on top.

Cooked carrots
3–4 carrots
1 dl vegetable broth
1 teaspoon almond puree
1 pinch each fruit sugar and sea salt
marjoram, thyme, rosemary, parsley

Cut the carrots in strips or rounds and cook in the vegetable broth for 30–45 min. Stir in the almond puree. Season and sprinkle with chopped parsley.

Peas and carrots
(As soon as the peas are tolerated; avoid with flatulence.)
½ tablespoon olive oil
100 g fresh peas, shelled
1 dl vegetable broth
marjoram, thyme, lovage
parsley, chives
150 g sliced carrots, prepared according to the above recipe for cooked carrots.

Briefly sauté peas in the olive oil, add vegetable broth and cook until soft. Season. Season. Mix carrots and peas, or serve separately.

Peas, French style
¼ head of lettuce or romaine lettuce
150–200 g peas, shelled
1 dl vegetable broth
1 pinch sea salt
parsley, chives marjoram, thyme, lovage
10 g nut spread
1 teaspoon wholegrain flour

Sauté the lettuce or romaine lettuce cut into fine strips with the peas in the vegetable broth over very low heat until soft. Season. Mix nut spread with wholegrain flour, add and boil briefly.

Cooked sugar peas (snow peas) (mange tout)
(Diet-stages IV–V.)
200 g snow peas
1 dl vegetable broth
1 pinch sea salt
1 pinch sugar (Succanat)
a little parsley or lovage
chives, marjoram, thyme
fresh butter, olive oil or nut spread

Cook sugar peas and herbs covered in the vegetable broth for ½ to ¾ hour. Season and add fresh butter, olive oil or nut spread when serving.

Green beans with tomatoes
(Avoid at first if suffering from meteorism.)
(Diet-stages IV–V.)
250 g beans
a little garlic
savoury, parsley
1–2 tomatoes
1 pinch sea salt
some caraway, marjoram, lovage

Sauté the beans, finely diced tomatoes and herbs for approx. 1 hour. Add water if necessary. Season to taste.

Steamed celery root (celeriac)
½ celery root (celeriac)
1 dl vegetable broth
1 pinch sea salt
lemon juice, marjoram
1 teaspoon almond puree
very thin slices of apple, nuts

Pour vegetable broth over the julienned celery root (celeriac) and cook until soft, ½ to ¾ hour. Season. To refine, add almond puree and, if desired, apple slices. Sprinkle with chopped nuts.

Celery root (celeriac) with béchamel sauce
Prepare 1 small celery root (celeriac) as described above and mix with Béchamel sauce (see recipe page 87).

Beetroots
Cut off the root tips and leaves to approx. 2 cm and wash thoroughly without damaging the skin.

350 g beetroots
1 dl vegetable broth
1 pinch each fruit sugar and
1 pinch sea salt
¼ laurel leaf, lovage, caraway, nutmeg
touch of garlic, parsley
lemon juice, lemon balm
1 tablespoon wholegrain flour, mixed cold
1 tablespoon almond puree

Cook the beetroots soft in the pressure cooker for approx. 25 min. Peel and cut into thin slices. Mix thoroughly with the herbs and spices in the vegetable broth and cook over low heat for 15 min. To bind, stir in the wholegrain flour and finally add the almond puree.

Jerusalem artichoke
250 g Jerusalem artichoke
a little vegetable broth
1 pinch sea salt
basil
1 teaspoon almond puree

Cook the Jerusalem artichoke like jacket potatoes (see recipe page 82). Peel, slice and cook until soft in the vegetable broth. Season and add the almond puree to refine.
You can also prepare the Jerusalem artichoke with béchamel sauce (see recipe page 87) and grated cheese.

Stewed tomatoes
4–5 tomatoes
½ tablespoon olive oil
½ onion
1 teaspoon fruit sugar
1 pinch sea salt
touch of garlic
rosemary, marjoram, basil
1 tablespoon corn starch (optional)
parsley or chives or dill

Slightly brown onion and fruit sugar in olive oil in the pan. Douse the tomatoes with boiling water, then peel them, cut them into pieces, add them to the onions and cook the mixture until it has thickened a little. Add garlic and spices and finish cooking (add corn starch to thicken). Sprinkle plenty of chopped parsley or other herbs on the prepared tomatoes.

Steamed tomatoes
2–3 tomatoes
1 pinch sea salt
10 g olive oil or butter

¼ onion, chopped
a pinch of herbes de Provence (basil, rosemary, thyme, sage) parsley

Sauté the onion without fat. Put the halved tomatoes on a greased tray or oven-proof dish. Rub olive oil on each tomato half, and spread the sautéed onion and herbs on it. Cook briefly in the oven. Some tomatoes may be blended or very finely chopped, blended with cream, heated quickly and spread on the prepared tomato.

Stuffed tomatoes
2–3 tomatoes
1 teaspoon rice per tomato
1 pinch sea salt
olive oil or nut spread
a little onion and garlic
rosemary, marjoram, thyme, basil
bay leaf, nutmeg
vegetable broth (optional)

Cut out the top of the tomatoes and hollow out the core. Chop the tomato pulp and mix with 1 teaspoon uncooked rice and the herbs and spices. Fill in the core with the mixture, add olive oil and replace the tops of the tomatoes Bake in the oven at a good bottom heat for 20–30 min.

Tomatoes à la provençale
2 tomatoes
1 pinch sea salt
1 tablespoon chopped parsley
1 tablespoon breadcrumbs

Halve tomatoes, sprinkle sea salt on them and place on a tray. Mix breadcrumbs and parsley and spread on the tomatoes with a spoon. Bake in the oven for 15 min.

Courgettes with tomatoes
½ tablespoon olive oil
½ onion, chopped
300 g courgette
50 g tomato
1 pinch sea salt

garlic, rosemary, marjoram, thyme, basil
parsley, chives, dill
maize flour (optional)
1 teaspoon almond puree

Simmer onion in olive oil. Dice the courgettes, peel and dice the tomatoes. Add the vegetables to the onions and cook them until soft. Season. If there is too much liquid, add stirred-up maize flour and 1 teaspoon almond puree before serving.

Sweet peppers (green, yellow, red)
These are very suitable as additions to other dishes.
(for low-acidic stomachs, not acidic irritable stomachs.)
150–200 g sweet peppers
½ tablespoon olive oil
½ onion, chopped
1 pinch sea salt
garlic, rosemary, marjoram, thyme, basil, parsley

Cut the sweet peppers in strips and sauté them in olive oil with the onion, herbs and spices in a covered pan for at least ½ hour.

Ratatouille
(Not for acidic irritable stomachs.)
50 g sweet peppers
100 g courgette
50 g aubergine
1 tomato
½ onion, chopped
a little garlic
1 tablespoon olive oil
1 pinch sea salt
rosemary, marjoram, thyme, basil, parsley

Chop the sweet peppers, courgettes, aubergines and tomato (peeled). Sauté onion and garlic in olive oil, add vegetables and cook covered for 1 hour. Season. If there is too much sauce, let it thicken while uncovered.

Aubergines
Wash the aubergines, peel (optional)
1 teaspoon olive oil
400–500 g aubergines
a little vegetable broth (optional)
sea salt

Steam the aubergines, cut into cubes, and sauté in olive oil until soft, add salt. Garnish with a few tomato halves or with stewed tomatoes.

Artichokes
1 artichoke
¾ l water
1 tablespoon lemon juice
1 pinch sea salt

Cut off the stalks close to the artichokes. Remove the bottommost hard leaves and remove the tips. Halve and cut out the heart; wash under running water and rub the cut surface with lemon juice. Let water come to the boil, add lemon juice and sea salt and cook the artichoke until soft for approx. ¾ h. Drain and serve the artichoke on a warm platter covered with a serviette. Serve with yoghurt sauce (see recipe page 67).

Asparagus
½ bunch of asparagus
1 l water
1 pinch sea salt
grated cheese
nut spread

Wash the asparagus and peel the stalks thoroughly. Green asparagus can be left almost whole. Cook the asparagus in boiling water until soft for 20–30 min. (green asparagus take much less time), remove with a slotted skimming spoon and serve on a platter covered with a serviette. Sprinkle grated cheese and pour liquid nut spread over the dish. As a variation, serve with vinaigrette sauce (see recipe page 89).

Cauliflower or broccoli
(Do not use if suffering from flatulence.)
(Only from organic production.)
1 small cauliflower or broccoli (250 g)
1 teaspoon olive oil
1 garlic clove
1 dl vegetable broth
1 pinch sea salt, pepper
pine nuts or almond slices

Cut off the leaves and stalk below the florets. Peel the stalk and cut into larger pieces; divide the flower into florets. Lightly brown the chopped garlic clove in olive oil, add the cauliflower or broccoli and sauté briefly. Douse with the vegetable broth and then cook for approx. 5 minutes. Season with salt and pepper. Briefly roasted pine nuts or sliced almond without fat in a pan and spread on the vegetables.

Kohlrabi with herbs
(Avoid at first if suffering from meteorism.)
(Diet-stage V only.)
1 kohlrabi
1 dl vegetable broth
1 tablespoon tender kohlrabi leaves, chopped
béchamel sauce (see recipe page 87)

Cut kohlrabi into 4 pieces then into fine slices. Cook covered in the vegetable broth for ½–¾ hour. Add the kohlrabi leaves and cream before serving. Mix the béchamel sauce with chopped herbs and pour over the cooked kohlrabi.

Brussels sprouts, steamed
(Avoid if suffering from meteorism!)
(Only from organic production and only in stage-V diet.)
½ tablespoon olive oil
200 g Brussels sprouts, cleaned
1 dl vegetable broth
1 pinch sea salt
nutmeg, basil

Slightly sauté Brussels sprouts in olive oil. Add vegetable broth and continue cooking for ½ hr until soft. Season. Add a little liquid nut spread when serving (optional).

Cabbage* or white cabbage, steamed
(Avoid if suffering from meteorism.)
(All cabbage types must be chewed well. Only in stage-V diet is raw cabbage juice always permitted! See note.)
½ tablespoon olive oil
½ onion, chopped
250 g young cabbage
1 dl vegetable broth
a little Kelpamare (optional)
nutmeg, caraway, 1 pinch sea salt,
basil or lovage

Sauté onions in olive oil. Cut cabbage in strips 2 cm wide, add to the onions and cook until the vegetables begin to soften. Add vegetable broth and cook over low heat for ½ hr. until soft. Season. Green, mature cabbage must be blanched briefly before cooking.

Cabbage chopped*
(Avoid if suffering from meteorism.)
(Stage IV diet only.)
200 g cabbage
1 dl water
½ tablespoon olive oil
a little garlic
1 small tablespoon flour
1 dl vegetable broth or half milk, half vegetable broth
1–2 tablespoons cream
Kelpamare, nutmeg, caraway, parsley
1 pinch sea salt

Cut the cabbage into 4 pieces, cook until soft, drain and chop finely. Sauté briefly in olive oil, sprinkle with finely chopped garlic and flour, and cook for ¼ hour. Add vegetable broth or milk and heat. Season. Enrich with cream.

Red cabbage*
(Avoid in meteorism.)
(Stage–V diet only.)
½ teaspoon olive oil
250 g red cabbage
½ teaspoon lemon juice
½ apple
½ teaspoon rice
1 dl vegetable broth
½ dl grape juice or fruit juice
1 apple
a little butter
1 pinch sea salt

Steam the finely grated red cabbage in olive oil. Add lemon juice, apple cut into fine slices, and rice. Continue steaming. Add vegetable broth and grape juice or fruit juice and steam until soft, covered over low heat for 1–1½ hours. Peel the second apple, cut into wedges. Add butter and braise the apple wedges on a tin baking sheet in the oven. Garnish the prepared red cabbage with the apple wedges.

Leeks
(Avoid if suffering from meteorism.)
(Stage II diet only.)
200 g leek, cleaned and prepared
½ tablespoon olive oil
1 dl vegetable broth
½ tablespoon cream
1 pinch sea salt
grated cheese (optional)

Cut leeks into 10 cm pieces and layer them in the pan. Add olive oil and vegetable broth and cook slowly while covered. After cooking, add salt and cream and sprinkle with grated cheese (optional).

Salads of cooked vegetables

Carrots, celery, beetroot, beans, cauliflower, broccoli, courgettes, mangold and Swiss chard are particularly suitable for these salads.

The vegetables are cooked until soft in vegetable broth or water, drained and cut small (diced, sliced, florets, strips). Serve with salad dressing or with vinaigrette or mayonnaise. Use onions and chopped herbs to enhance.

Potato salad
(Only in the regular diet)
200 g potatoes
½ dl vegetable broth
1 tablespoon mayonnaise (see recipe page 67, 88)
½ tablespoon chopped onions
borage, chives, parsley, lemon balm, marjoram, thyme, dill

Cook the potatoes soft in the pressure cooker, peel while hot, and slice. Pour the heated vegetable broth over them and let stand for a bit, then mix in the mayonnaise. Season with onions and herbs. Mayonnaise can be replaced with oil, lemon juice and cream well mixed and added to the potatoes.

Potato salad with cucumbers
(If cucumbers are tolerated!)
1 large potato
¼ cucumber
2 tablespoons yoghurt sauce (see recipe page 67)
½ garlic clove
dill or borage, chives, parsley, onion

Prepare the potato as described above. Grate the peeled cucumber with a coarse grater and add to the potato. Mix with yoghurt sauce and season with onions and herbs.
Rub the salad bowl with the garlic clove before serving.

Salade niçoise
1 boiled potato
1 small tomato
radishes
several cucumber slices
1 hard-boiled egg
1 tablespoon olive oil
½ tablespoon lemon juice
1 pinch sea salt
parsley, chives or dill,
lemon balm, borage
a few leaves of head lettuce

Slice the potato, tomato, radish and egg and, together with the cucumber slices, add a salad dressing of oil, lemon juice, sea salt and herbs. Just before serving, cut the leaves of head lettuce into broad strips and mix with the salad, or prepare the salad on the head lettuce leaves.

Rice salad
50 g rice
2 dl water
2 tablespoons quark dressing (see recipe page 67)
½ tablespoon chopped onions
¼ tomato
chives, parsley or basil
a few salad leaves

Cook the rice in water, rinse it briefly and let it cool. Add the onion, finely diced tomato and herbs to the quark sauce.
Mix the rice with the dressing and prepare on salad leaves.

Celery root (celeriac) salad with soy mayonnaise
½ small celery root (celeriac)
½–1 tablespoon lemon juice
2 walnuts
¼ apple (optional)
1 pinch sea salt
1 tablespoon soy mayonnaise (see recipe page 67, 88)

Cut the raw celery root (celeriac) into match-thin strips or grate it. Add lemon juice to prevent browning. Add the coarsely chopped walnuts and the grated apple and mix with the mayonnaise.

Vegetable aspics
2½ dl vegetable broth
2 g agar-agar
drops of lemon juice
Kelpamare
fresh slices of cucumber
cubes of tomato
broccoli flowers, cooked
peas, cooked
beans, cooked and finely chopped

Agar-agar is a plant-based gelatine powder that is used for vegetable and fruit aspics, sauces and puddings, etc. instead of animal gelatine.
Add agar-agar powder to the lukewarm vegetable broth and heat slowly until the gelling agent is thoroughly dissolved. Season with lemon juice and Kelpamare. Pour a little aspic into the rinsed moulds and let it harden. Garnish with vegetable slices, add more aspic, let it harden and repeat until the moulds are filled.
Turn over the cooled aspics and serve on salad leaves.

Potato Dishes

Jacket potatoes
3–4 small potatoes
water

Brush and wash potatoes. Fill pan with steamer insert or wire screen with water up to the insert, add potatoes, cover and cook for 30 to 40 minutes. (8–10 minutes in the pressure cooker.)

Baked potatoes
3–4 small potatoes
1 tablespoon olive oil
butter or nut spread

Brush and wash the potatoes. Score the peel 3–4 times, brush with oil and bake them on a greased sheet at medium heat for 30–40 min. Put a dab of nut spread on each of the cooked potatoes.

Quark potatoes
3–4 small potatoes
50 g low fat quark
1–2 tablespoons milk or cream
chives or caraway or marjoram
1 pinch sea salt

Make a shallow cut into the top of the potatoes and prepare them as for baked potatoes. For the stuffing, stir quark with milk or cream until smooth and add seasonings. Use a spoon to spread into the shallow cut of the baked potatoes or apply with a piping bag.

Caraway potatoes
2–3 medium-sized, longish narrow potatoes
1 teaspoon caraway
1 pinch sea salt
1 tablespoon olive oil

Wash and clean the potatoes and cut them in half crosswise. Mix caraway with sea salt and sprinkle on the cut side of the potatoes. Place the potatoes with the cut side down on a greased tray, brush with olive oil and bake at medium heat for ¾ hour.

Bouillon potatoes
250 g potatoes
1–2 dl vegetable broth
1 pinch sea salt
lovage, thyme
10 g butter or olive oil or nut spread

Wash potatoes, peel, halve or cut into pieces and cook until soft in the vegetable broth with the sea salt and spices. Spread butter or olive oil or nut spread on the prepared potatoes.

Cream potatoes
200 g potatoes
onion, chopped
1 dl vegetable broth
1 pinch sea salt
½ dl cream or milk (optional)

thyme, nutmeg,
parsley

Peel, slice and briefly sauté potatoes and onion without fat. Cook until soft with the vegetable broth and spices. Add cream or milk before serving. Sprinkle the prepared potatoes with chopped parsley.

Potatoes with tomatoes
200 g potatoes
½ small onion
1 dl vegetable broth
1 small tomato
1 pinch sea salt
1 tablespoon cream or sesame cream (see recipe page 70)
Marjoram, rosemary or thyme

Briefly sauté the chopped onion and peeled, sliced potatoes without fat, then cook them in the vegetable broth until semi-soft. Cut the peeled tomato into wedges, add and finish cooking. Season. Add the cream or sesame cream before serving.

Mashed potatoes
4 potatoes
dried tomatoes
butter or olive oil or nut spread

Wash, peel, quarter and steam the potatoes until soft. Rice the potatoes onto a warm plate. Add liquid butter or olive oil or nut spread and garnish with minced dried tomatoes.

Potato puree
4 potatoes
1 dl milk
nutmeg
1 tablespoon cream (optional)
1 pinch sea salt
finely chopped marjoram and caraway
garlic
dried tomatoes

Peel and slice the potatoes and steam them until soft. Strain through the potato ricer. Heat milk, add the potato mash, stir until smooth and season. Add cream if desired. Serve on a hot platter, garnished with minced dried tomatoes.

Potato dumplings
4 potatoes
1 dl milk
10 g butter
10 g butter or nut spread
1 pinch sea salt
nutmeg

Prepare mashed potatoes as described above. Dip a small ladle in liquid butter, cut out dumplings and serve on hot platter, dressed with butter or nut spread.

Roast potatoes
2 small potatoes
1 pinch sea salt
1 dl vegetable broth
1–2 tablespoons cream or sesame cream (see recipe page 70) or nut spread
nutmeg, thyme, parsley
Peel and halve potatoes and steam them until semi-soft. Put them on an ovenproof platter with the cut side down. Cover with vegetable broth. Season and roast in the oven until the liquid has thickened. Add cream or nut spread and continue roasting until the potatoes are lightly browned. Serve with the cut side facing up and sprinkle with chopped parsley.

Potato slices with spinach
1 large potato
1 dl vegetable broth
1 pinch sea salt
100 g spinach
butter, olive oil or nut spread
garlic, parsley, chives
peppermint, sage or nutmeg (optional)

Cut the peeled potato lengthwise into slices 1 cm thick and cook carefully until soft. Place on a buttered tray. Prepare the spinach like leaf spinach (see recipe page 74), season and distribute over the potatoes. Sprinkle with grated cheese if desired and brush with butter or olive oil or nut spread. Bake briefly in the oven.

Potato goulash
(Not for irritable stomach.)
1 onion
1 large potato
1 green sweet pepper
1–2 dl water
1 pinch sea salt
marjoram, thyme, rosemary, parsley

Finely dice the onion and potato, julienne the sweet pepper and cover with water in a pan. Cook until soft, approx. 15 minutes. Season well and serve.

Ayurveda potatoes
(An attractive, aromatic dish that yields 3–4 helpings.)
5 large potatoes
½ soy drink
1 package of soy crème (substitute for crème fraîche)
1 bunch each of fresh dill, fresh chives and fresh parsley
juice of ½ lemon
1–2 teaspoons turmeric
½ teaspoon curry
soy sauce

Cut the cleaned potatoes into thick slices and cook them for approx. 5 minutes. In the meantime, slowly heat the soy drink in a pan, mixed with the soy crème (do not boil). Stir in turmeric and curry to taste and season with soy sauce. Put the potato slices in the sauce and simmer for approx. 10 minutes. Sprinkle the fresh, finely chopped herbs on the potatoes and serve at once.

Cereal Dishes

Japanese rice
80 g wholegrain rice
1½–2 dl vegetable bouillon
1 pinch sea salt
10 g butter or olive oil or nut spread
1 small peeled onion studded with clove and bay leaf

Put the rice in the cooking bouillon with the studded onion and boil for 40 minutes. Let cool and remove the onion. Reheat the rice in the oven and top with heated butter or olive oil or nut spread before serving.

Risotto
80 g wholegrain rice
1 tablespoon chopped onion
2 dl vegetable broth or water
1 pinch sea salt
dried mushrooms
fresh herbs to taste
rosemary
10 g fresh butter or olive oil
or nut spread
10 g Parmesan cheese (optional)

Sauté the rice with the onion until the rice is translucent. Add the vegetable broth or hot water and cook until al dente (30–40 minutes). Add the finely chopped, dried mushrooms and herbs and cook briefly together. Before serving, mix in butter or olive oil or nut spread and grated Parmesan cheese with a fork.

Saffron rice
Prepare like risotto. Dissolve a knife tip of saffron powder in a little bouillon and add to rice.

Riz creole with vegetables
½ tablespoon olive oil
80 g wholegrain rice
2 tablespoons dices of vegetables (leeks, celery, carrots)
2 dl vegetable broth

1 pinch sea salt
freshly chopped herbs to taste

Briefly sauté rice and vegetables, add hot vegetable broth and herbs and cook for 30–45 min.

Tomato rice
80 g wholegrain rice
1 tablespoon chopped onion
a little garlic, pressed
1 large tomato
approx. 1 dl vegetable broth
1 pinch sea salt
rosemary, marjoram, nutmeg,
optional basil
whole-cane sugar (Succanat)
10 g butter or olive oil

Sauté onion, garlic and rice until the rice is translucent. Add peeled, diced tomato. Add vegetable broth and spices and cook for 30–45 min. Add fresh butter or olive oil before serving.

Rice with courgettes
½ tablespoon olive oil
80 g wholegrain rice
1 tablespoon onion, chopped
150 g courgettes
1 pinch sea salt
1½ dl vegetable broth or water
freshly chopped dill
10 g butter, olive oil or nut spread

Diced the courgettes. Prepare dish as for tomato rice (see above)

Rice with spinach
(Only if spinach is allowed.)
80 g wholegrain rice
100 g spinach
some onion, chopped
2 dl vegetable broth or water
1 pinch sea salt
nutmeg and peppermint
10 g fresh butter, olive oil or nut spread

Cut spinach coarsely. Prepare dish as for tomato rice (see above).

Risi bisi (rice with peas)
80 g wholegrain rice
150 g tender peas, shelled
some onion, chopped
1 pinch each of fruit sugar and sea salt
½ dl vegetable broth
1½–2 dl water
10 g butter or olive oil or nut spread
parsley

Sauté onion with fruit sugar and sea salt. Add the peas and cook briefly, then add vegetable broth and cook the peas until soft. Prepare risotto (according to the above recipe) in a separate pan. Add the peas to the cooked risotto. Before serving, top the prepared rice with butter or olive oil or nut spread and chopped parsley.

Rice gratin with tomatoes
½ tablespoon olive oil
80 g wholegrain rice
2 small tomatoes
some onion, chopped
2 tablespoons vegetables (leek, celery, carrots)
1½ dl vegetable broth
1 pinch sea salt
parsley, lovage
5 g butter or olive oil

Briefly sauté onion and very finely diced vegetables, add the rice and continue cooking until translucent. Douse with hot vegetable broth, season and cook for 30–45 min. Put the finished rice and the sliced tomatoes into an oven-proof mould in layers, top with dabs of butter or brush on olive oil, and bake in the oven for 10 min.

Indian rice dish
80 g wholegrain rice
2 dl vegetable broth
1 pinch sea salt
1 small banana

1 small apple
1 tablespoon raisins
1 teaspoon sunflower seeds
1 teaspoon sesame seeds
saffron, curry, fresh ginger root

Cook rice with vegetable broth and 1 pinch of sea salt until not quite soft (approx. 30–40 minutes). Mix the sliced banana, the peeled and sliced apple, and the raisins into the rice and continue boiling for 5–10 min. Season with saffron, curry and ginger root to taste. Sprinkle with sunflower seeds and lightly dry-roasted (without fat) sesame seeds.

Semolina mash
50 g semolina
3 dl milk
2 dl water
1 pinch sea salt
1 tablespoon sesame cream (see recipe page 70)
1 tablespoon each of fruit sugar and cinnamon

Stir semolina into the boiling liquid a, salt and cook for 15–20 min. Sprinkle the cream and fruit sugar mixed with cinnamon onto the prepared semolina mash.

Polenta
½ tablespoon olive oil
50 g maize semolina, medium fine
3 dl water
nutmeg
1 pinch sea salt
½ tablespoon fresh butter or
olive oil or nut meg

Oil the pan. Boil water and stir in the maize. Boil for 5 min. over low heat, stirring frequently. Season and continue boiling for 45–60 min. over low heat. At the end, mix in butter or olive oil or nutmeg. You may also add onion slices sautéed without fat.

Millet risotto
½ tablespoon olive oil
50 g millet
1 tablespoon chopped onion
1½ dl vegetable broth
½ onion
1 pinch sea salt

Sauté onion and hot-rinsed millet in olive oil until glazed, add the hot vegetable broth and salt and cook for 20 min. Before serving, top with julienned or sliced onion sautéed without fat.

Millet risotto with vegetables
40 g millet
1 tablespoon chopped onion
2 tablespoons finely chopped vegetable cubes
(leek, celery, carrots or carrots and peas)
1½ dl vegetable broth
Kelpamare
rosemary
1 tablespoon grated cheese (optional)
10 g fresh butter or nut spread

Sauté onion, diced vegetable and hot-rinsed millet until glazed. Add hot vegetable broth, season and boil for 20 min. Before serving, top with dabs of butter (optional) or dabs of nut spread.

Coarse-ground grain mash
2 tablespoons coarse-ground grain
(wheat, oats, rye)
3 tablespoons water
1 pinch sea salt

Soak the coarse-ground grain for 12 hours then boil in water for 10 min. or cook for ½ hour in a bain-marie. Salt.

Pasta, spaghetti, macaroni, etc.
For a strict healing diet, egg pasta should not be used. Today there also are high quality wholegrain pastas, soy pastas and spelt pastas in addition to well-known Italian pasta products made from wheat. Note that many sauces contain large

quantities of fat (oil, butter, cheese, cream).
The best-tolerated pasta products are cooked al dente with a classic or simple tomato sauce (see recipes page 88).

Spätzle or Knöpfli (without egg)
(Only in the regular diet.)
60 g wholegrain flour
20 g soy flour
1 dl diluted milk
1 l water
1 pinch sea salt
1 tablespoon olive oil
onion, julienned
chives and parsley

Mix wholegrain and soy flour thoroughly with diluted milk and tap the mixture until the dough forms bubbles. Let rest for at least 1 hour. Boil water with sea salt. Press the dough in portions through a coarse screen into the boiling water or put it onto a small wooden cutting board. Cut fine strips with a knife and place them in the boiling water. Let the Knöpfli or Spätzle simmer until they rise to the surface. Take them out with a skimmer and place them on a hot platter. As desired, garnish with julienned onion sautéed in olive oil (or without fat), chives and parsley.

Spinach or tomato Knöpfli
70 g wholegrain flour (⅓ soy flour)
1 egg
1 dl milk water
1 handful of chopped, raw spinach or
1 teaspoon tomato puree
1 dl water
1 tablespoon sea salt
chives and parsley

Make a smooth batter from the wholemeal and soy flour, egg and water, and let it rest for 1 hour. Prepare and cook like Spätzle according to the recipe above. Add spinach and tomato puree. Season with chives and parsley.

Sauces

Sauces are difficult for a healing diet, since almost all recipes contain large quantities of fat (butter, oil, cream), cheese and eggs. The combination of hot fat and flour (béchamel sauce) should always be avoided, because this mixture is very hard on the stomach, liver and intestines. We have put together a few adapted sauces here, whose recipes deviate from the classical ones. All of them taste great.

Classical béchamel sauce (recipe 1)
(As an exception in the regular diet.)
½ teaspoon olive oil
½ teaspoon butter
1 teaspoon flour
½ dl milk
½ dl vegetable broth or water
1 pinch sea salt, nutmeg
freshly ground white pepper

Heat butter and olive oil, sift in the flour and sauté slightly. Slowly add milk and vegetable broth while constantly stirring. Cook for 20 minutes. Salt and flavour.

Béchamel sauce without egg (recipe 2)
For 4 persons:
2–3 tablespoons wheat flour
1 l milk
1 bay leaf
1 tablespoon vegetable broth
1 grated onion
1 pinch each of sea salt, nutmeg and freshly ground white pepper
chopped parsley

Briefly cook the flour without fat until it is aromatic (it must not turn dark), then let cool slightly. Add the milk, bay leaf, vegetable broth and onion while stirring constantly. Bring to a boil. Season. After approx. 5 minutes, remove the bay leaf and serve the sauce sprinkled with parsley.

This basic sauce can be used to make many versions. For example:

Horseradish sauce
At the end, add 10 g finely grated horseradish and cook the sauce for another 5 min.

Caper sauce
Season the finished sauce with whole or chopped capers and lemon juice.

Olive sauce
Briefly cook the sauce with 4–5 tablespoons tomato pulp and 2 tablespoons chopped olives. Season with a knife point of cayenne pepper (optional).

Herb sauce
Mix plenty of finely chopped herbs such as parsley, lovage, chervil, basil, estragon, oregano, etc. into the finished sauce.

Champignon sauce
Mix 3–4 tablespoons of very finely chopped raw champignons into the finished sauce and season with lemon juice.

Béchamel sauce (recipe 3)
For 4 persons:
2 tablespoons wheat flour
½ l soy milk
1 bay leaf
1 onion, finely grated
2 teaspoons red miso
1 pinch each of pepper and paprika
chopped parsley

Briefly brown the flour without fat until it gives off a toasted aroma. Let cool a little, then add the soy milk while stirring constantly. Add the bay leaf and onion and boil for about 5 min.
Stir in the miso, remove the bay leaf and season the sauce with pepper and paprika. Sprinkle with chopped parsley. (Miso is a fermented soybean paste that is great for seasoning. It tastes like soy sauce but does not contain salt.)

Tomato sauce, classic
½ tablespoon olive oil
1 tablespoon onion
½ garlic clove, pressed
2 tablespoons carrot, celery, leek
2 small tomatoes
1 pinch sea salt
1 pinch raw-cane sugar (Succanat)
1 teaspoon tomato puree
1½ dl vegetable broth or water
bay leaf, rosemary, thyme

Sauté the chopped onion, pressed garlic and coarsely cut vegetables in olive oil. Add the diced tomatoes and the tomato puree, then add vegetable broth (or water). Season and simmer for ½ hour. Strain if desired.

Tomato sauce, simple
3 tomatoes
1 pinch each sea salt and raw-cane sugar (Sucanat)
chives, basil
1 tablespoon olive oil

Dice tomatoes, steam until soft, season and drain. Add olive oil to taste.

Mayonnaise, classic
(Only in stage-IV and stage-V diets.)
For 4 persons:
1 egg yolk
1 tablespoon lemon juice
2 dl olive oil
1 pinch sea salt
onion, herbs, Kelpamare

Mix the egg yolk well with several drops of lemon juice. Add the oil drop by drop while stirring evenly with the whisk. If the mayonnaise grows too thick, dilute with lemon juice. Season to taste.

Remoulade sauce, classic
(Only for stage-IV and stage-V diets.)
For 4 persons:
Prepare mayonnaise according to above recipe

1 hardboiled egg, chopped
1 tablespoon cornichons, chopped
some capers
1 teaspoon parsley, chopped
small tomato diced

Mix the various ingredients with the finished mayonnaise. Garnish with diced tomato.

Mayonnaise without animal protein
See recipe page 67.

Remoulade sauce without animal protein
For 4 persons:
Prepare mayonnaise without animal protein (see recipe page 67) and mix with
1 tablespoon chopped cornichons, capers and chopped parsley. Garnish with diced tomato.

Vinaigrette
For 4 persons:
2 tablespoons olive oil
2 tablespoons groundnut oil
2½ tablespoons lemon juice
2 tablespoons water or vegetable broth
½ onion, chopped
1 egg, hard boiled and chopped
1–2 cornichons, cut or finely chopped
parsley or chives
1 tablespoon small tomato, diced
1 pinch sea salt

Whisk olive oil, lemon juice and vegetable broth until smooth, then add the other ingredients, mixing thoroughly.

Sandwiches

Sandwiches are generally popular as appetizers, for a summer meal, to take along on hikes and journeys, and as lunch at the office.
Spreads and ingredients can be used in any number of ways, and various wholegrain bread types are available, some already pre-sliced.

The recipes are for 4 persons.

Basic spreads
For the strict diet, spread some quark on the bread rolls and add raw food.

Guacamole
2 ripe avocados
juice of ½ lemon
½ small onion, chopped
2 garlic cloves, pressed
sea salt and white pepper (optional)

Mash the removed flesh of the avocados with the lemon juice in a blender. Mix in onion and garlic and season with sea salt and white pepper. If desired, stir in 1 tablespoon soy cream (instead of crème fraiche).

Sweet avocado cream
1 ripe avocado
4 tablespoons fresh orange juice
1 tablespoon honey
1 knife tip ginger powder

Mash the removed pulp of the avocado by squeezing or blending and mix in the other ingredients. Serve at once.

Tofu spread with nuts
250 g tofu, pureed
2 finely chopped spring onions
50 g nuts (hazelnuts, walnuts, almonds, cashews)
1 pinch sea salt and white pepper (optional)

Lightly roast the nuts in the oven or a dry pan, let them cool and then grind them. Mix with the pureed tofu and onion. Season with sea salt and pepper.

Quark spread with herbs
100 g quark
10 g butter or nut spread
Kelpamare or miso
caraway, chives or herbs (dill, borage, lovage, basil, oregano, peppermint etc.)

Stir quark and vegetable margarine to a frothy consistency, season and add individual herbs (or a mix) for variety.

Garnishes
Spreads can be garnished in the following ways:
with raw carrots or celery
with tomatoes, fresh cucumbers, radish, cress, onion, nuts,
parsley, chives etc.

Desserts
The following recipes are for 4 persons.

Desserts should be eaten with great restraint. Use honey (acacia honey is particularly good), maple syrup, agave juice or whole-cane sugar (Sucanat, Panela, etc.), though the latter is not suitable for all sweet dishes because of its strong taste. Do not eat any sweet dishes with large quantities of sugar, eggs or cream. There are many tasty alternatives.

Fruit salad
2 tablespoons honey
1 dl water
1–2 dl grape juice or apple juice
1–2 tablespoons lemon juice
600 g apricots or peaches
melons
apples
pears (ripe)
red cherries, pitted
berries

Cook water with honey, grape juice and lemon juice and let cool. Thinly slice seasonal fruits and add them to the syrup.

Filled melons
2 small melons
fruit salad as per recipe above

Halve the melons, scoop out the seeds and fill the melons with the fruit salad.

Fruit jelly
3 dl water or grape juice
1–2 tablespoons honey
10 g agar-agar, powdered
7 dl orange or berry juice
Agar-agar is a plant-based gelatine powder that is used for vegetable and fruit spreads, sauces and puddings, etc. instead of animal gelatine.

Mix water, honey and agar-agar and cook over low heat while stirring constantly until the agar-agar has dissolved. Add fruit juice and serve immediately in glasses or desert cups. Garnish with sesame cream to taste (see recipe page 70).

Apple sauce
800 g apples
2 dl water or apple juice
1–2 tablespoons honey
cinnamon or lemon peel
1 dl sesame cream (see recipe page 70)

Core and cut the apples into pieces, cook them in the water or apple juice and honey until soft, and strain them. Mix with cinnamon or lemon peel (from untreated lemons). To enrich, serve sesame cream with the apple sauce.

Apple or pear compote
800 g apples or pears
2–3 dl water or apple juice
1 tablespoon honey
grated lemon peel (from untreated lemons)
or cinnamon

Core and peel the apples or pears, and cut them into wedges. Bring water or juice to a boil, add honey and lemon peel or cinnamon, add the fruit, and cook until soft.

Baked apples (recipe 1)
800 g apples
½ l water or apple juice
1 tablespoon honey

¼ cinnamon stick
quince, raspberry or currant jelly
(see recipe page 90)
or raisins and wine berries with a little honey

Boil water or apple juice with honey and cinnamon stick. Peel, core, halve and place apple portions in the hot water or juice. Cook slowly until soft. Remove with skimmer and place on a flat platter with the cut surface up. Fill the apples with jelly or mix of raisin, wine, berry and honey.

Baked apples (recipe 2)
4 large or 8 small apples
4 tablespoons ground hazelnuts
2 tablespoons currants
4 tablespoons sesame cream (see recipe page 70)
1–2 tablespoons honey
grated lemon peel (untreated lemon)
10 g butter or nut spread
1 tablespoon whole-cane sugar
1–2 dl apple juice

Mix hazelnuts, currants, sesame cream, honey and lemon peel, fill the prepared apples (cored and peeled) and place the apples in a casserole. Add butter or nut spread and sugar and pour 1 cm. apple juice over the apples. Bake for 20–30 min.

Dried fruit salad with grapes and pine nuts
200 g dried figs
200 g dates
200 g dried apples
400 g white grapes
juice of 1 lemon
2 tablespoons honey
50 g pine nuts

Chop the dried fruit, halve one half of the grapes and squeeze the others. Put all fruits in a dish. Mix the lemon juice and grape juice with the honey and pour it over the fruits. Cool before serving. Toast the pine nuts and sprinkle them over the fruit salad.

Blueberry mash (Heitisturm)
(Slightly constipating.)
1 kg blueberries
80–100 g fruit sugar
2 dl water
1 tablespoon flour
2 tablespoons water
30 g butter or nut spread or almond spread
20 g bread cubes

Wash the blueberries and cook them with water and fruit sugar for 5–10 minutes. Stir the flour into a little water, add, cook and prepare. Slightly toast the bread cubes in butter and add to the blueberries.

Strawberry or raspberry cream
300 g berries
vanilla cream
1–2 dl cream or sesame cream (see recipe page 70)

Prepare a vanilla cream according to the recipe on page 132 and mix with the mixed or pureed berries. Fold in cream or sesame cream or serve separately.

Lemon cream
¾ l milk
1–2 lemons, untreated
1 tablespoon cornflour or arrowroot flour
3 tablespoons milk
2 tablespoons honey
cream or sesame cream (see recipe page 70) to taste

Slice lemon peel thin and boil in the milk. Add cornflour or arrowroot flour stirred with a little cold milk and honey and boil briefly. Add more honey and return to the pan, stirring constantly, and heat almost to a boil. Strain the cooled cream and add a few spoons of lemon juice and sesame cream to taste.

Orange cream
Prepare as lemon cream
(See recipe above.)

Orange aspics
5 dl orange juice
5 g agar-agar, powdered vegetable jelly instead of gelatine
1 tablespoon fruit sugar

Mix thoroughly 3 dl orange juice, agar-agar and sugar and heat over a low flame while stirring constantly (do not boil) until the agar-agar has dissolved completely. Add the remaining orange juice and pour it into chilled moulds. Let cool.

Sesame bars
100 g Syramena sugar
2 tablespoons honey
100 g sesame seeds, whole not ground

Syramena sugar is a light raw cane sugar available in health-food stores. Heat the sugar in a dry pan and stir until a light caramel forms. Add the liquid honey and mix well. Add the sesame and mix well again. Pour the mass into a mould or onto an oiled board, let cool slightly and cut into squares or diamonds. Let cool.

Vanilla sauce/cream
1 vanilla pod
¼ l water
40 g wheat flour
3 tablespoon honey
approx. 200 ml soy milk

Split the vanilla pod lengthwise, scrape the seeds into the water, add the pod and bring to a boil. Put the wheat flour into the vanilla water while stirring constantly and let it swell into a thick mash. Let it cool a little, then stir in the honey and soy milk. Depending on the amount of soy milk, you will get vanilla crème or vanilla sauce. Keep cool until serving.

Almond milk sauce
4 dl milk
50 g almonds or almond spread
2 tablespoons honey
1 tablespoon cornflour
or arrowroot flour
2 tablespoons water

Boil milk with the peeled, ground almonds (or the almond spread) and honey. Stir cornflour or arrowroot flour in cold water and stir into the boiling milk. Mix the finished sauce.

Rosehip sauce
70 g rosehip puree or rosehip pulp
2 dl water or grape juice
1–2 tablespoons honey
a few drops of lemon juice (optional)

Boil the ingredients together, then add the lemon juice.

Red wine sauce
2 dl water
lemon or orange peel (untreated fruits)
1 cinnamon stalk
1 clove
1–2 tablespoons honey
2 dl red grape juice
20 g almonds

Boil water, peel, spices and honey together for a few min., then strain. Add grape juice and heat (do not boil). Add peeled and sliced almonds.

Red fruit jelly (chilled soup)
7 dl currant, raspberry or strawberry juice
3 dl red grape juice or water
70 g semolina
1 tablespoon cornflour

Boil berry juice and grape juice together, stir in semolina and cornflour and boil for 10 min. Pour into rinsed pudding mould and cool.
Serve with vanilla sauce (see recipe

page 92) or almond milk sauce (see recipe page 92).

Red fruit jelly, Danish style
1 kg berries (raspberries, currants, strawberries or pitted cherries, or all mixed)
1 l fruit juice (e.g. elderberry)
2 packs of agar-agar
honey to taste
½ teaspoon natural vanilla
sesame cream, liquid (see recipe page 70)

Put cleaned and chopped (optional) fruits into a dish, mix with honey and vanilla. Heat the fruit juice with agar-agar and pour the liquid over the fruits. Let the fruit jelly harden.
Serve with liquid sesame cream.

Suggestion for menus Sorted according to Different Consistency Types

For their application, see p. 52 **'DIETS' juice** type **(diet II).**

a) Day's menu for a juice day in bed or fruit-juice fasting day
a) Strict form: 600 g juice.
8 AM: 200 g fruit juice, unsweetened, freshly made of grapefruit, oranges, tangerines, berries, peaches, melons, etc. Possibly mixed with cereal gruel.
12.30 PM: 200 g fruit juice (as above) or 200 g fresh vegetable juice (e.g. carrots, tomatoes, spinach, beetroot), mixed or pure, with a few drops of lemon juice.
6 PM: 200 g fruit juice as at 8 AM.
Condition: strict bed rest, weight and urine control after 24 hours. Duration 1–3 days, longer only under medical supervision.
In case of strong thirst or if the urine quantity is insufficient (less than 800 ccm in 24 hours), 1–3 cups of 150 g rose hip tea or other teas can be drunk additionally.
b) Milder form: 800 g juice.
8 AM: 200 g fruit juice.
12 PM: 200 g mixed or pure vegetable juice.
4 PM: 200 g fruit juice (changing composition).
8 PM: 150–200 g carrot or tomato juice.
Condition: Duration and application as in the strict form.

b) Day's menu of a full juice day
Breakfast 200 g fruit juice (gruel-cream addition as prescribed, pectin agar-agar) 150 g almond milk or soy milk or yoghurt 1 cup rose hip tea with honey (optional)
Lunch 200 g fruit juice 150 g almond milk or sesame milk (Helva or yoghurt) 150 g vegetable juice of different kinds or mixed from 2–3 types
Dinner 200 g fruit juice 150 g almond milk or yoghurt

If fat must be almost entirely removed, the milk share can be given in the form of buttermilk, low-fat plain yoghurt or whey.

Pureed Type (Diet III)
c) Raw diet day in pureed form
Breakfast 200 g mixed muesli or strained 150 g fruit juice 150 g almond milk 1 cup tea
Lunch 200 g fruit juice 150 g almond milk mixed raw vegetables comprising tomatoes, lettuce, carrots
Dinner same as breakfast

d) Raw diet with addition, pureed
Breakfast Same as in section c above.
Lunch 150 g fruit juice 150 g almond milk 150 g vegetable juice or mixed raw vegetables: tomatoes, lettuce, celery 200 g vegetable bouillon mashed potatoes
Dinner see pureed raw diet

e) Transition diet, pureed
Breakfast   250 g mixed muesli
150 g fruit juice
1 cup herbal tea, or milk, or yoghurt
1 Darwida and butter and honey
or 1 crisp bread or wholemeal rusk
Lunch   150 g fruit juice
150 g mixed raw vegetables
cooked foods: green spelt soup, strained
lettuce, chopped
mashed potatoes
Dinner   250 g mixed muesli
cooked food: cereal soup
herbal tea

Bland healing diet (diet IV)
f) Raw food day in refined form
Breakfast   muesli, strained (optional)
150 g almond milk or pine nuts or finely ground almonds
150 g fruit juice, rose-hip tea (optional)
Lunch   150 g fruit juice or finely crushed fruits (berries, peaches, bananas etc.)
raw vegetables (beets, finely grated, zucchini, chopped, head lettuce, chopped)
almond milk or pine nuts
Dinner   same as breakfast.

g) Raw food with addition in refined form
Breakfast   same as in section f above.
Lunch   150 g fruit juice or finely crushed fruits
raw vegetables: horseradish, finely grated
cooked foods: spinach, finely chopped, tomatoes, finely chopped
200 g vegetable bouillon
bouillon potatoes
Dinner   see raw food in refined form (plus 1 piece of crispbread, optional)
cooked foods: spinach, finely chopped

h) Transition diet in refined form
Breakfast   250 g muesli
Lunch   150 g fruit juice or finely crushed fruits
raw vegetables: black salsifies, finely grated, endives, finely chopped, tomatoes, finely chopped
cooked foods: potato soup, strained
fennel, finely chopped
risotto
Dinner   150 g fruit juice
1 cup herbal tea, or milk, or yoghurt
1 crisp bread with butter

Protective diet of different types Diet V:
fruit fasting – raw food– raw food with additions – transition diet

1) Fruit Fasting
Fruit fasting may replace juice fasting in bed (the strict form of the fruit juice fasting day), e.g. when metabolism change and stimulation of the intestine with cellulose content is the principal aim rather than protection due to omission of cellulose. Since this diet produces a strong feeling of satiation, fruit fasting can be performed even on days without complete rest, and for extended periods of time. The effect of juice fasting is, however, more intense.

Fruit fasting is indicated for persons with a lazy intestine (apple, banana or blueberry day) and accumulation of food in the abdomen. Duration 1–5 days, longer if medically prescribed. Can also be used for weight reduction.

Daily menu: 2 times 200–250 g washed, fresh, fully ripe unsweetened fruit.

Special fruit fasting types
Apple day: 5–6 times 1 large apple finely ground for acute gastrointestinal catarrh with diarrhoea.

Strawberry day: 3–4 times 200–250 g very ripe strawberries, unsweetened.

Blueberry day: 3 times 200–250 g blueberries. Mildly constipating, mildly cleansing.

Blackberry day: 3 times 200–250–300 g blackberries. Particularly rich in natural sugar and vitamin C. Nutritious and easy to digest.

Currant day: 3 times 200–250 g (⅔ red and yellow, ⅓ black) currants. Rich in vitamin C. Particularly refreshing and thirst-quenching for liver patients.

Japanese-persimmon day: 2 small (or 1 large) Japanese persimmon (kaki) fruits, 4 times a day. Very nutritious and rich in vitamins C and B.

Grape day (traditional grape treatment): 750–1000 g grapes, eaten over 4–5 meals per day. Wash thoroughly and clean of treatment residue. Eat the entire fruit. Low in vitamins, but particularly nutritious because of its high, easily absorbable fruit-sugar content. Liver protection! Stimulates intestine with seeds. Duration: 1–2 weeks, longer if prescribed by doctor (up to 6 weeks).

Fig day:
3 times 200 g fresh figs. Stimulates the intestine. Nutritious. No more than 1 day.

k) Raw food day in the normal form
Breakfast	muesli
	fruits (all fruits except for apricots and plums)
	pine nuts, hazelnuts, almonds
Lunch	fruits
	raw vegetables: cauliflower, tomatoes, lettuce
	pine nuts, hazelnuts, almonds
Dinner	same as breakfast

l) Raw food with addition
Breakfast	same as in section k
Lunch	fruits
	raw vegetables: Chinese cabbage, beetroots, almonds, hazelnuts
	cooked foods: zucchini 200 g vegetable bouillon, baked potatoes
Dinner	see raw food in normal form (plus 1 crispbread or Darwida)

m) Transition diet in normal form
Breakfast	same as in section k
Lunch	fruits
	raw vegetables: cress, cucumbers, small carrots
	cooked foods: vegetable bouillon
	rice gratin with tomatoes
Dinner	fruits
	1 cup herbal tea, or milk, or yoghurt
	1 piece of wholemeal bread with butter

Menu for 1 week of permanent diet
1st day
Breakfast	250 g muesli
	1–2 piece of wholemeal bread
	10 g butter
	honey or quark (optional)
	fruits
	herbal tea
Lunch	fruits
	raw vegetables: celery, dandelion, head lettuce
	cooked foods: beetroots
	quark potatoes
	pear compote

Dinner yoghurt with fruit salad
or muesli
sandwiches
or whole rice and head lettuce or meal mash with cream

Breakfast and dinner of the following days as on the 1st day.

2nd day
Lunch fruits
raw vegetables: black salsifies, radicchio, endives (chicory)
cooked foods: cream of rice soup
halved tomatoes with scrambled egg
hirsotto

3rd day
Lunch fruits
raw vegetables: beetroot, white cabbage, head lettuce
cooked foods: artichokes with butter sauce
Swiss chard with tomatoes
potato mash

4th day
Lunch fruits
raw vegetables: cauliflower, tomatoes, head lettuce
cooked foods: small carrots
spinach heads
strawberry chilled soup

5th day
Lunch fruits
raw vegetables: radish, spinach, head lettuce
cooked foods: tomato soup, sugar peas (snow peas, mange tout)
cream potatoes

6th day
Lunch fruits
raw vegetables: fennel, small carrots, head lettuce
cooked foods: lettuce
riz creole
junket with raspberries

7th day
Lunch fruits
raw vegetables: kohlrabi, tomatoes, head lettuce
cooked foods: zucchini
polenta
apple sauce

Summary of the Foods for the Healing Diet for Digestive Problems*

1. Anti-inflammatory and calming in case of overstimulation of the stomach and intestine (see diet II–A)
Wholemeal gruels (pure or mixed with fresh juices), **agar-agar, pectin,** barley, whole rice. Specially note **whole wheat gel** (Dr. Kousas) which, prepared as a 'gel' of whole wheat, has an outstanding nutritional and calming effect on gastrointestinal mucosa. Together with chopped fruits, or fruit juices or raw vegetables (raw vegetable juices), and spices and sour milk, this gel is a complete bland diet in contrast to the old-fashioned white-flour-mash bland diet. It has a simultaneously detoxifying, diuretic and flatulence-inhibiting effect. Gel food, 50 g, combined with the above mentioned fresh food, can be consumed (cooked with water for 1 min.) 4 to 5 times per day as a one week treatment. However, it is not suitable for Herter patients (coeliac disease). **Healing earth** (clay for internal use)* between the meals with water or calming herbal teas. **Potato juice, cabbage juice, certified raw milk** in sips. First class **fresh cream,** low-fat **cheese,** without salt. **Whey cheese,** fresh, non-sour buttermilk, whey, junket, chamomile tea.

2. Appetite stimulation, invigoration of the digestive juices (see 106 and diet II–C p. 52)
Yeast products, herbal **spice, sea salt** instead of table salt, **soy spice. Vegetable bouillon** (vegetable bouillon cubes), **herbal quark** and cheese. **Kitchen herbs:** marjoram, tarragon, dill, aniseed. **Bitter vegetables:** cardon, chicoree. **Raw vegetable juices spiced with herbs**, for working persons and if no juicer is at hand: 100 % natural plant juices in bottles. **Sourdough breads, grains, flakes, nuts, raisins, berries, citrus fruits,** sweet-tart **apple, bitter tea, centaury tea.**

3. Intestine stimulating for constipation (see p. 59, 106)
Wholemeal dishes such as meal mash, sprouted grains, wholemeal bread and wheat gel. **Cereal gruels** with slightly laxative effect, such as flax**seed** ground or whole (cooked to gruel with water), **flea seeds** (psyllium) soaked, **fresh fruit, fresh vegetables** (green), **dried fruit** (especially figs, plums, pears), **rhubarb, yoghurt, sour milk, whey, sauerkraut** or sauerkraut water, **sourdough breads.**

4. Constipating effect for diarrhoea (see diet II–C)
Apple, banana, blueberry juice fresh, blueberries dried, **healing earth** (clay for internal use), **carob flour, rice gruel,** flour, **dry rice, tormentil** tea, **blackberry leaf tea.**

5. Flatulence inhibiting (see p. 26)
Healing earth, yoghurt, buttermilk, whey, flatulence tea (fennel, caraway, aniseed), flax**seed gruel, whole wheat gel. Marsh drinking treatment.** Avoid: cooked cabbage (instead, eat it raw or consume as a juice), confectionery and sweet milk!

---

* The herbal teas for gastrointestinal patients are described in detail in the chapter 'Types of Diet' and the recipe section. Or moor-mud drinking treatment.

6. Food for convalescence

Minerals, effective substances, vitamins: sea salt, wholemeal cereals, all fresh vegetables (juice or whole) and fruits, sea buckthorn whole fruit, wild herb extracts (stinging nettle, birch, watercress, etc.), sprouted cereals.

Raw cane sugar and starch: wholemeal flour, flakes, meal, bread, wheat sprouts or wheat sprouted at home, wholemeal rusks, pumpernickel, crispbread, Darwida, sourdough bread, fruit sugar syrup, honey, fruit concentrates, naturally cloudy fruit juices, grape juice, raw icing sugar (of sugar cane), all sweet fruit, carrots, beetroots.

Whole fat: cold-pressed sunflower, flaxseed, poppy oil, grain sprout oil, first-class, uncoloured. Fresh butter and cream, unhydrogenated vegetable fats as bread spread. Pine nuts, almonds, brasil nuts and other nuts. Sesame products.

Whole protein (lactovegetarian): soy products (bread spread, flour, flakes), almond and hazelnut products (puree, milk, bread spreads), sesame products. Sour milk, buttermilk, yoghurt. Whey. Junket, lean milk, certified raw milk. Lean and whole quark with addition of herbs, salt, honey. Soft cheese. Salt-free cheese. Whey cheese. Raw, fresh egg with fruit juice, whisked or in soup. (Diet table, see page 104.)

Indications for General Applications for Gastrointestinal Disease

Stomach over-acidification	Cold abdominal wash in the evening, or in the morning, or at night; steam compress over the liver or the stomach.
Flatulence	Abdominal wash, steam compress, alternating warm and cold foot baths, hip baths, hot Priessnitz body compress, cold body wash, body compress, cold half bath, alternating foot bath, lower abdominal wash
Digestion problems	Thigh gush, lower abdominal gush, Kuhne friction hip bath (rectum), cold half bath, body wash, alternating foot bath, abdominal wash, Kneipp steam compresses.
Stimulation of the entire digestive system	Kuhne and Priessnitz body compresses.
Colic	Full wash, Kneipp steam compress.
Constipation	Lower abdominal wash, Kneipp steam compress.

Baths

Kuhne's friction hip bath

Indication
Diseases and weakness of the pelvic organs (bladder, sexual organs, women's complaints, prostate complaints, rectal complaints).

First, sit in a hot hip bath, with the lower legs on a stool placed in the bathtub so that only your pelvis is in the water.

Then empty the bathtub, sit on the stool, place a bucket of cold water in front of you and apply cold water to the inside of your thighs and perineum repeatedly by slapping with a cold bath towel submersed in the bucket of cold water. Start above the knees and treat your thighs moving upwards eventually to the perineum. There should be a strong reddening of the skin and pleasant inner warming. Then lie in bed wrapped warmly.

Alternating foot bath

Indication
Bile duct inflammation, jaundice, cold feet, sleeping problems, flatulence.

Place 2 large buckets next to each other, fill one with very warm water, the other with very cold water, and sit in front of them.
First submerse your feet and lower legs in the warm water for 5 minutes, then the cold one for 10–15 seconds. Put feet into warm stockings at once and rest covered warmly.

Cold half-bath
(according to Winternitz, Kuhne, Kneipp)

Indication
Gallstones, sleeping problems, digestion problems, flatulence, constipation.

After thorough warming, slowly enter the bath tub and sit in the cold water, which should reach your navel. Inhale deeply. Stay in the cold water for 6–10 seconds (later increase gradually to 1 minute), dry off thoroughly at once and lie down covered warmly to rest. According to Dr Winternitz, this bath, supplemented by a **moving** cold gush of the abdomen, improves portal-vein circulation.

Washes

Cold abdominal wash

Indication
Flatulence, digestion problems.

Lie on the bed and rub your abdomen with a cold wash cloth or a cold and wet hand, in a clockwise direction, for 2–3 minutes.
Rest covered warmly.

Full wash

Indication
Improves defences, regulation of weakness of the circulation and the heat balance, promotes skin circulation and stimulates the inner organs, for chronic rheumatic diseases, nervousness and sleeping problems.
For bile-duct inflammation or jaundice, we recommend adding vinegar (expansion of the skin vessels) with 1 part vinegar to 2 parts water (according to Dr. Spengler).

Procedure
Outside and inside the right arm to the armpit, repeat on the left, then throat, chest, body, back, right leg outside and inside, then behind, from the buttocks down; repeat on the left; finally soles of both foot in sequence.
This wash should be carried out quickly, and the rag should be put back into the cool water repeatedly. Do not dry off right away (evaporation coldness). Then dry off briskly and rest covered warmly.

Body wash

Indication
Digestion problems (intestinal inertia, flatulence), problems falling asleep, Caution: for bladder infections, use the overheating bath.
You should first be quite warm.

Prepare a tub with cold water and a terrycloth rag. Start with the moist rag in the area of the appendix and rotate it to below the breast in a clockwise motion 20–40 times. Remoisten the rag several times. Then rest covered warmly.

Lower abdominal wash

Indication
Intestinal inertia, flatulence.
Caution: for urinary tract infection use the overheating bath.
Proceed as for the body wash but wash only the abdomen.
Then rest covered warmly.

Abdominal wash

Indication
Flatulence, digestion problems.

Lie on a pre-heated bed and wash your abdomen with a wash cloth dipped in cold water, rotating it clockwise approx. 50 times. Dip the wash cloth into cold water regularly.
Rest warmly covered.

Cold gushes (Kneipp, Winternitz)

Thigh gush

Indication
Regulation problems of the circulation (orthostatic circulation weakness), varicose diseases, problems falling asleep, digestion problems.

Proceed as for the full body gush, but treat only the legs.
End the gush with the sole of the foot on both sides.
The thoroughly warmed patient stands in the tub or shower with his back to the water jet. The helper sprays a weak, wide water jet on the patient: starting at the back of the right foot, quickly up the outside of the leg to the buttocks and back down to the heel on the inside. Then the left leg is treated in the same manner. End the gush with the sole of the foot (both sides).

The abdominal gush according to Winternitz

Indication
Digestion problems, abdominal problems, prostate conditions.

This treatment increases and expands the stimulation of the leg gush.
It is performed the same way, but the insides of the thighs are treated for longer and the jet stays on the abdomen for approx. 8 seconds.
The general previous heating is particularly important here. Lie down afterwards and wrap yourself warmly. This will stimulate the pelvic organs wonderfully.

Compresses

Kuhne and Priessnitz body compresses

Indication
Stimulation of the entire digestive system and the liver in liver diseases, metabolism problems, digestive problems, flatulence, constipation, sleeping problems, menopausal complaints, nervousness.
on the bed
First place a woollen blanket that should reach from the neck to the feet. Place a 1 m wide rubber or plastic cloth above it crosswise.

Now fold a linen cloth to 1 × 2 metres and place it across the woollen blanket. This is the envelope for the compress. It should reach from the armpits to the knees. If the blankets are not pre-heated (tumbler dryer), the patient should lie on them and fold them around himself until they become warm. Now open the blankets again. The patient sits up or gets out of bed briefly
The actual compress cloth should be approx. 160 × 180 cm (linen is better than cotton). It is folded to 80 cm and put in cold water, wrung out briefly and quickly spread across the cotton blanket in the middle. The patient lies on it at once so that the cloth reaches from his armpits to the groin. The legs are placed together and the arms are held up. He should now inhale and briefly hold his breath (this makes the cold stimulus feel pleasant.). Fold in the compress cloth and then the dry cotton cloth closely and without rucks around the patient at once. Place his arms along his sides. Now the patient is closely wrapped in the woollen blanket from the armpits to the feet and covered in a warm blanket. The entire procedure must be performed quickly.
Let the patient rest for 1½–3 hours like this with the window opened. If he falls asleep, you can also leave the compress on much longer, but no longer than until it has become hot and dry.

Compresses and applications

Kneipp steam compress

Indication
This treatment relaxes the muscles. Colic and cramps of inner organs, flatulence, liver-gallbladder pain, digestion problems or muscle tension.

Procedure
A folded linen cloth of suitable size is submersed in boiling water (caution:

danger of burns). The cloth is taken from the water with a tool, placed in terrycloth, wrung and folded in a flannel cloth for a compress, which is placed on the area to be treated when it is no longer considered too hot on the upper arm, and wrapped up, fastened with an elastic bandage. Once the compress has cooled, it is removed. This should be followed by at least one hour of bed rest.

Massages

Belly massage (Winternitz method)

Indication
Constipation from intestinal inertia, flatulence.

The patient lies relaxed on the back or the left side. Start on the right abdomen and continue the massage clockwise along the course of the large intestine to the left abdomen. Reach into the abdominal wall gently but deeply with both hands and slowly massage the abdomen.

Diet Table for Patients with Gastrointestinal Diseases

I. Tea fasting (for p. 52)
150–1000 g herbal tea (5–6 glasses with 150 g). Tea types: chamomile – linden blossom – peppermint – rose hip – blueberry – blackberry leaves – strawberry leaves – flaxseed – tormentil – wormwood tea. mixed herbal teas: flatulence tea, bitter tea. (For preparation and use of the various tea types, see recipes on page 62)
During tea fasting, maintain bed rest at consistent warmth until the acute complaints have subsided. – Duration: according to doctor's orders

	II. Juice diet (see p. 52)	III. Mash diet (for p. 56)	IV. Bland healing diet, convalescence (for p. 58)	V. Protective healing diet for disease prevention (for p. 59)
Fruit	All fresh fruit juices (pure or mixed with cream or ⅓ cereal gruel or in almond milk, whisked in banana or in apple or in pectin-agar heads	II, III + grapes (thoroughly washed), Birchermuesli (normal), II + all fruit types mixed as fresh mash, carefully chosen high-quality organically grown ripe fruit chosen according to individual needs (caution: pesticides), Birchermuesli, mixed; cooked: compotes (strained, little sweetening)	II, III + grapes (thoroughly washed), Birchermuesli (normal or with yoghurt or cream)	I, II, III + all ripe fresh fruit (chew well), exceptionally, cooked compotes a
Vegetables	Raw, juices of all types (mixed with ⅓ cream or gruel or naturally in juice press or from centrifugal juicer); cooked: homemade (natural) vegetable bouillon	II + raw vegetables (mixed = puree), all types of cooked vegetables (strained), cabbage (not permitted at first) later permitted	II, III + raw vegetables (finely chopped with oil, lemon, cream, herbs); cooked: steamed, all types, chosen according to tolerance	II, III, IV + all vegetables (raw and cooked, chew well, quality: organically grown if possible, well cleaned, do not pour off water, do not reheat), fresh butter or oil (for steaming or freshly for preparation)

* Do not use any gluten-containing cereals in Herter patients (wheat, rye).

	II. Juice diet (for p. 52)	**III. Mash diet (for p. 56)**	**IV. Bland healing diet convalescence (for p. 58)**	**V. Protective healing diet disease prevention (for p. 59)**
Sugar	Honey (dissolved in tea and juices), raw icing sugar (dissolved), fruit concentrates (dissolved)	As II (mixed into fruit mash and muesli)	As II + fruit concentrates, common raw cane sugar	As in IV, white sugar as an exception; do not eat chocolate or candy
Starch (cereals, potatoes)	Cereal gruels (flaxseed, barley, oats, rice, wheat, ⅓ mixed with juices or pure)*, wheat gel (grain), (Gastrikur)	Whole cereal flakes in muesli or milk, cereal soups, cereal grouts, mashes, crisp bread (well chewed)*, potato puree, mashed potatoes	Crispbread, pumpernickel, Darwi-da, wholemeal breads, wheat sprouts (grains, sprouted), rice, corn, millet, whole cereal meals and. grouts*, all potato foods	Wholemeal bread, meal mash, sprouted wheat, all cereal foods, wholemeal flours, wholemeal pasta*
Fats	Vegetable oils (cold-pressed), flaxseed, sunflower, olive oil), cream (fresh, moderate amounts!)	As II, butter, nut butter, fine margarine (moderate amounts)	As II + III	As II + III, rarely with roasted, baked foods, heated fats (no hydrogenated fats)
Proteins	Vegetable: Almond, soy, sesame milk, raw vegetable juices Animal: milk, yoghurt, organic yoghurt, buttermilk, whey, beaten egg yolk (now and then)	II + veg.: for crème, bread spread, flakes, milk: Hazelnut paste and almond puree, sesame, soy; Animal: Quark, Milk mashes and shakes, quark crèmes, junket	II, III + all milk types (veg. and animal), wholemeal cereal*, rarely egg dishes, cheese (very mild)	As IV + quark-fruit crème, cheese (diff. types, mild), quark with herbs, eggs (2 per week), meat (up to 2 times per week if desired)
Drinks	Fresh, fruit and vegetable juices, vegetable bouillon (nature), all milk types (almond, soy, sesame milk), herbal teas (see recipes), fruit concentrates according to individual wishes (diluted), mineral water (uncarbonated)	Same as II	Same as II, with apple juice, sterile grape juices, cooled juices (not iced; drink slowly)	Same as II–IV, no alcohol, no coffee, no black tea
Spices	Sea salt in vegetable bouillon and gruels	Same as II, mild kitchen herbs optional	Same as II + fresh kitchen herbs (rosemary, thyme, dill, lovage, marjoram, tarragon, balm), vegetable and yeast extracts	Same as IV, according to personal taste also a little nutmeg, a little sweet pepper (spice mildly)

* Do not use any gluten-containing cereals in Herter patients (wheat, rye).

The following effects specifically apply:

	Stimulating gastric juices, appetite stimulating	**Calming gastric juices**	**Stimulating the intestine (for constipation)**	**Calming the intestine (for diarrhoea and flatulence)**
Fruit	Citric fruits, ripe, not overly sweet grapes, all berries, melons, sweet, ripe peaches, plums, cherries	Apple, banana, juices in ⅓ gruel or pectin-agar aspics, grape juice (sweet, mild)	Citrus fruits, berries, grapes, rhubarb, drupes (ripe), dried fruit (figs, plums)	Blueberry compote (dried and fresh blueberries), blueberry juice or tea, strawberry, blackcurrant, apple (grated), banana
Vegetables	All raw vegetables (chewed well), particularly spinach, cress, sauerkraut (raw and cooked)	Raw juices + cream 1 teaspoon + gruel ⅓ + potato juice (raw); mixed or in juice: particularly carrots, beetroots and cabbage	All raw vegetables, cooked vegetables (chewed well)	Raw vegetables as juice (no spinach and cabbages), cooked vegetables (pureed, no spinach)
Sugars	Honey, fruit concentrates and Stevia	–	Honey and fruit concentrates, Stevia, raw and cane sugar	–
Starch (cereals, potatoes)	Wholemeal cereal (sprouted), grains, meal, grouts, wholemeal bread, (sourdough), boiled potatoes in skins and baked potatoes	Rice-barley-oats gruel (mashed, salt-free), wheat gel (Kousa), cereal flakes and wholemeal mashes (with milk or water), (Gastrikur), crispbread D, mashed potatoes and juices (raw)	Wholemeal cereal (sprouted), wholemeal breads, meal, grouts, flaxseed meal and gruel, jacket potatoes and baked potatoes	Same as in 'calming gastric juices'
Fats	Vegetable oils (cold-pressed, small amount!)	Small amount: almond milk, cream, vegetable oil	Same as in 'Stimulating gastric juices'	Same as in 'calming gastric juices'
Proteins	Yoghurt, organic yoghurt, fruit milk (cold, mixed), sour milk, herbal cheese and quark, caraway cheese, etc.	Sweet milk, certified raw milk, almond milk, junket, quark (natural), mild soft cheese (Gervais, Petit-Suisse, Gala, etc.)	Same as in 'Stimulating gastric juices'	Same as in 'Calming gastric juices'
Drinks	Bitter tea, peppermint tea, centaury tea, rose hip tea, vegetable bouillon, fresh juices, apple juice and grape juice (sterilised), yoghurt, buttermilk, juniper juice, (sterilis, in spoonfuls)	Salt-free, natural, no spices	Cascara bark (*Cascara sagrada*) as spice or tea, small doses, flea seed (Psyllium), sea salt	Blackberry leaf tea, blueberries (dried, decoction), tormentil tea, balm tea, chamomile tea, orange blossom tea, peppermint tea, 'flatulence tea' (of caraway, fennel, aniseed)

	Stimulating gastric juices, appetite stimulating	Calming gastric juices	Stimulating the intestine (against constipation)	Calming the intestine (against diarrhoea and flatulence)
Spices	Salt-free, natural, no spices	Cascara bark (Cascara Sagrada, as spice or tea, small doses), flea seed (Psyllium), sea salt	–	Dried blueberries (well chewed)

List of Recipes

Appetite-stimulating food	98
Bland healing diet (diet IV), menu	95
Butter, pant fats and cooking, steaming/sautéing	70
Cereal Dishes	84
Constipating effect for diarrhoea	98
Continuous diet, menu for 1 week	96
Desserts	90
Diet Table	104
Dressings	66
Flatulence-inhibiting food	98
Food for convalescence	99
Foods and their effects on the digestion	47
Fresh juices	52, 61
Fruit Fasting	95
Full juice day	94
Healthful Teas	62
Inflammation-inhibiting food	98
Intestine stimulating for constipation	98
Juice fasting in bed	94
Juices	61
Menu for 1 week of permanent diet	96
Menus sortetd by different consistency	94
Milk Types	70
Muesli	63
Potato Dishes	82
Protective diet (diet V), menu	95
Raw food day, menu	95
Raw food day, normal form	96
Raw food day with addition	95
Raw vegetables and salads	65
Salad dressings	66
Salad dressing table, what fits	69
Salads	65
Salads of cooked vegetables	80
Sandwiches	89
Sauces	87
Soups	71
Teas	62
Transition diet in refined form	95
Transition diet, menu	96
Transition diet, pureed	95
Vegetable oils	70
Vegetables	74
Wholesmoe fat	99
Wholesome protein	99
Wholesome sugar	99

Notes

1 Bircher, A., *Bircher-Benner Handbuch für Leber- und Darmkrankheiten*, Edition Bircher-Benner, Braunwald, 32nd edition, p. 11, ISBN 9782970072225.
2 Sonnenburg, J.L. et al., 'Getting a grip on things: how do communities of bacterial symbionts become established in our intestine?', *Nat Immunol*.5, r. 6, 20014 pp. 568–573. PMID 15164016.
3 Wilson, M., *Microbial Inhabitants of Humans: Their Ecology and Role in Health and Disease*, Cambridge University Press, Cambridge, 2005, ISBN 0-521-84158-5.
4 Eckburg, P.B. et al., 'The role of microbes in Crohn's disease', *Clin. Infekt. Dis.* 2007, 44: 256–262.
5 Vieira, L.Q. et al., 'Parasitic infections in germfree animals', *Braz J Med Biol Res*, January 1998, Column 31(1)105–110.
6 Rakoff-Nahoum, S. et al., 'Intestinal flora and immune system', *Cell Biology* 2004: 118: 229–241.
7 Chung, H. et al., 'Immune maturation depends on colonization with a host-specific microbiota', *Cell Band* 149, Number 7, June 2012, S. 1578–1593, ISSN 1097–4172, doi: 10.1016/j. cel I 2012.04.037 PMID 22726443, PMC 342780.
8 Wolin, M.J. et al., 'Carbohydrate fermentation in human intestinal microflora in health and disease', Hentges D.J. (Ed.) Academic Press Inf., New York, USA 1983.
9 Ley, R.A. et al., 'An obesity associated gut microbiome with increased capacity for energy harvest', *Nature* Dec 2006, 21, 444(7122): 10 27–31.
10 Bäckhed, F. et al., 'Mechanisms underlying the resistance to diet-induced obesity in germ-free mice', *Proc Natl Acad Sci U S A* 2007 Jan 16, 104 (3): 979.84, Epub 2007 Jan 8.
11 Bäckhed, F. et al., 'The gut microbiota as an environmental factor that regulates fat storage', *Proc Natl Acad Sci U S A* 2004 Nov 2, 101(44): 15718–23, Epub 2004 Oct 25.
12 Barrett, N.R., 'The lower esophagus lined by columnar epithelium', *Surgery* 1957, 41: 881–894 PMID 13442856.
13 Cook, M.B. et al., 'A systematic review and meta-analysis of the sex ration for Barrett's esophagus, erosive reflux disease, and non-erosive reflux disease', *Am J Epidemiol* 2005 Dec 1, 162 (11): 1050–61 PMID 16221805.
14 Ronkainen, J. et al., 'Prevalence of Barrett's esophagus in the general population: an endoscopic study', *Gastroenterology* 2005 Dec, 129(6): 1852–31 PMID 16344051.
15 Sharma, P. et al., 'Relative risk of dysplasia for patients with intestinal metaplasia in the distal esophagus and in the gastric cardia', *Gut* 2000, 46: 9–13. 8, Dec 2006, PMID 1727775.
16 Coyle, M., 'Lifestile, genes, and cancer', *Methods Mol Biol* 472, 2009, 25–56 PMID 19107428.
17 *European Code Against Cancer and scientific justification*, 2 July 2003.
18 Deutsches Krebsforschungszentrum DKFH, Heidelberg, *Grundlagen der Krebsentstehung und Metastasenbildung*, 'Was ist Krebs?', April 2011, consulted on 4 Sept. 2014.
19 Khan, M. et al., 'Lifestyle as risk factor for cancer: evidence from human studies', *Cancer Lett* 293, 2010 133–143, PMID 2080335 (Review).
20 American Institute for Cancer Research/World Cancer Research Fund: 'Food, Nutrition, Physical Activity and the Prevention of Cancer', Internet-Archive, Version 27.2.2008, 2nd edition, 2007, ISBN 0–972-25222-3 93–94.
21 Boffetta, P., 'Fruit and Vegetable Intake and Overall Cancer Risk in the European Prospective Investigation into Cancer and Nutrition (EPIC)', *J Natl Cancer Inst* 102, 2010 429–537, doi: 10.1093/jnci/diq 072 PMIS 20371762.
22 World Health Organization WHO: *IARC Working Group on the Evaluation of Cancer-Preventive Agents*, IARC (editor) Band 6, IARC-Handbooks of Cancer Prevention, 2002, ISBN 9-283-23006-X.

23 Friedrich, C.M., 'Physical activity and cancer prevention: from observational to intervention research', *Cancer Epidemiol Biomarkers Prev* 10, 2001, 287–301, PMID 11319168.

24 Woods, J.A. et al., 'Effects of exercise on the immune response to cancer', *Med Sci Sports Exerc* 26, 1994, 1109–1115, PMID 7808244.

25 Woods et al., 'Exercise and cellular innate immune function', *Med Sci Sports Exerc* 31, 1999 57–66 PMID 9927011.

26 Pederen, P.K. et al., 'NK cell response to physical activity: possible mechanism of action', *Med Sci Sports Exerc* 26, 1994, S. 140–146, PMID 8164530.

27 Hoffmann, W. et al., 'Helicobacer pylori und gastroduodenale Ulcuskrankheit', *U Gastroenterol* 2009, 47, 68–102.

28 Piper, F., *Innere Medizin*, Heidelberg, 2007, 350–355.

29 Herold, G. et al., *Innere Medizin*, Köln, 2009, 418–421.

30 Liu, Chen et al., 'The gastrointestinal tract', *Pathologic Basis of Disease*, Vinag, Kumar et al., 7th edition, Philadelphia, 2005, 823–826

31 Thomas, C., *Histopathologie*, Stuttgart, 2006, p. 139.

32 Nato, J.M. et al., 'Iron deficiency accelerates Helicobacter pylori-induced carcinogenesis in rodents and humans', *The Journal of Clinical Investigation* Band 123, No. 1 Jan 2013, 1, pp. 479–492, ISSN 1558–8238.

33 Mitros, F. et al. 'The gastrointestinal tract', *Rubin's Pathology*, Raphael, Ruin et al., 5th edition, Philadelphia 2008, p. 569.

34 EPIC Symposium, Berlin, 'Was schützt vor Krebs und Diabetes? Konsenserklärung MMW-Fortschr', *Med*. No. 24/2007 (149 jg) p. 16, 25.4.2007.

35 Xie, F. et al., 'Coffee consumption and risk of gastric cancer: a large updated meta-analysis of prospective studies', Free *PMC* Article Sept 2014 18, 6(9), 3734–46, doi: 10.3390/nu6093734 PMID: 25237829 and PMCID: 4179186.

36 Sanikini, H. et al., 'Total, caffeinated and decaffeinated coffee and tea intake and gastric cancer risk: results from EPIC cohort study', *J Cancer* 2014 18 Sep 18, doi: 10.100.

37 Watzel, B et al., *Bioaktive Substanzen in Lebensmitteln*, Hippokrates-Verlag, Stuttgart, ISBN 3-7773-1115-41995.

38 Oynlola, O. et al., 'Fruit and vegetable consumption and all-cause, cancer and CVD mortality: analysis of health survey for England data', *J. Epidemiol Community Health*, Published Online first 19 April 2014, doi: 10.1136/jech-213–203500.

39 Steinmetz, et al., 'Vegetables, fruit and cancer II. Mechanisms Cancer Causes control 2', 1991 b, 427442.

40 Mayer, R., 'Gastrointestinal tract cancer', *Harrison's Principles of Internal Medicine*, volume I, New York, 2008, 571–573.

41 Huber, W. et al., 'Akute Pankreatitis, Evidenzbasierte Diagnostik und Therapie', *Deutsches Ärzteblatt* 104, No. 25, 22 June 2007, 1832–1842.

42 MacMahon, B. et al., 'Coffee and Cancer of the Pancreas', *N Engl J Med* 1981, 304: 630–633, March 1981, doi: 10.1056/NEJM198103123041102.

43 Vazquez-Roque, M. et al., 'A controlled trial of gluten-free diet in patients with irritable bowel syndrome-diarrhea: effects on bowel frequency and intestinal function', *Gastroenterology* volume 144, No. 5, May 2013, S. 903–911, E3, ISSN 1528–0012, Doi: 10.1053/j. gastro. 2013.01.049, PMID 23347715.

44 Pimentel, M., *A new IBS solution: bacteria – the missing link in treating irritable bowel syndrome*, Health Point Press, 2005.

45 Coutts, J. et al., *Management of Food-Allergens*, Wiley Blackwell, ISBN I.4051-6758-0 pp. 157 et seq.

46 Keller, R., Klinische Symptomatik, 'Zöliakie, ein Eisberg', *Monatsschrift Kinderheilkunde*, Heidelberg 151, 2003, 706–714, ISSN 0026–9298.

47 Rubio, A. et al., 'Increased prevalence and mortality in undiagnosed celiac disease', *Gastroenterology*, Col.137. No. 1, 2009, 88–93, ISSN 00165085, doi: 10.1053/j. gastro. 2009.03.059.

48 Kagnoff, M.F., 'Celiac disease: pathogenesis of a model immune-genetic disease', *J Clin Invest* 2007, 117(1): 41–49.

49 Riemann, J.F., *Gastroenterologie: das Referenzwerk für Klinik und Praxis*, 2007, Georg Thieme Verlag, ISBN 978.3-13-141201-0, p. 681.

50 Kiple, K.F., 'Lactose Intolerance', *Cambridge World History of Food*, edited by Keneth F. Kipple, Cambridge 2000, p. 1060.

51 Kretchmer, N., 'Lactose and Lactase', *Scientific American*, Oct. 1972, Michael de Vrese et al.

52 Leiss, O., 'Diätetische Therapie bei Kohlenhydratmalabsorption und Laktoseintolernaz', *Aktuel. Ernähr. Med.* volume 30, 2006, 75–87.

53 Muir, S.I.G., Review of 'Fructose malabsorption and the bigger picture', *Aliment Pharmacol Ther.* 252007, pp. 349–363.
54 Ramessen, J.J. et al., 'Absorption capacity of monosaccharides', *Gut.* 27, 1986, 1161–1168.
55 Truswell, A.S. et al., 'Incomplete absorption of pure fructose in healthy subjects and the facilitating effect of glucose', *Am J Clin Nutr.* 48, 1988, 1424–1430.
56 Born, P. et al., 'Colonic bacterial activity determines the symptoms in people with fructose-malabsorption', *Hepato-Gastroenterology* 42, 1995, 778–785, PMID 8847022.
57 Caspary, F.W., 'Diarrhoea associated with carbohydrate malabsorption', *Clinics in Gastroenterology* 15, No. 3, 1986, pp. 631–655.
58 Smith, P.J. et al., 'Introduction to metabolic activities of intestinal bacteria', *Am J Clin Nurt.* 32, 1979, 149–157.
59 Choy, F.C. et al., 'Fructose intolerance: an underrecognized problem', *Am J Gastroenterol* 2003, 98 (6) 1348–1353.
60 Ledochowski, M. et al., 'Fructose malabsorption and the decrease of serum tryptophan concentration', G. Huerther et al., *ISTRY 98 Proceedings: Tryptophan, Serotonin, Melatonin – Basic aspects and applications,* Plenum Press, New York, London, 1999, 73–78.
61 Nucera, G. et al., 'Abnormal breath tests to lactose, fructose and sorbitol in irritable bowel syndrome may be explained by small intestinal bacterial overgrowth', *Aliment Pharmacol Ther.* 21, 2005, 1391–1395.
62 Coutts, J. et al., *Management of food allergens*, Blackwell-Wiley, ISBN 1-4051-6758-0 pp. 157 et seq.
63 Jarisch, R., *Histaminintoleranz, Histamin und Seekrankheit*, 2 Aufl Georg Thieme-Verlag, Stuttgart New York, 2004, ISBN 3-13-195382-8 p. 15.
64 Baumgart, D.C. et al., 'Inflammatory bowel disease: cause and immunobiology', *Lancet* 169, No. 9573, 1627–1640.
65 Baumgart, D.C. et al., 'Crohn's disease', *Lancet* 2012, doi: 10.1016/SO140-6736(12)60026–9 PMID 22914295.
66 Jacobsen, B.A. et al., 'Increase in incidence and prevalence of inflammatory bowel disease in northern Denmark: a population-based study', 1978–2002, *Eur J Gastroenterol Hepatol*, 2006 June, 18(6), 601–606 PMID16702848.

67 'Pressekonferenz zum Crohn- und Colitistag 2011: Neue Erkenntnisse zur Ursache von chronisch entzündlichen Darmerkankungen', 15 Sept 2011, Leipzig.
68 Fellmann K. et al., 'A chromosome 8 gen cluster polymorphism with low human β-defensin 2 gene copy number predisposes to Crohn's disease of the colon', *Am J Hum Genet* 79 (2006) 39–448.
69 'Europäisches Institut für Lebensmittel- und Ernährungswissenschaft: Morbus Crohn durch Mycobakterien: ein Verdacht wird zur Gewissheit', 2/2009, 21–24.
70 Van Assche, G. et al., 'The second European evidence-based consensus on the diagnosis and management of Crohn's disease: definitions and diagnosis', *J Crohns Colitis*, volume 4 No. 1, Feb 2010, 7–27 ISSN 18764479.
71 Baumgartner, D.C. et al., 'Inflammatory bowel disease, clinical aspects and established and evolving therapies', *Lancet* 169, No. 9573, 2007, 1641–1657, Doi: 10.1016/SO140-6736(07)60751-X. PMID 17499606.
72 Rembacken, B.J. et al., Non-pathogenic Escherichia coli versus Mesalazine for the treatment of ulcerative colitis: a randomized trial, *Lancet*, 1999 Aug 21, 354(9179); 635.639 PMID 10466665.
73 Kruis, W. et al., 'Maintaining remission of ulcerative colitis with the probiotic Escherichia coli Nissle 1917 is as effective as Mesalzine Gut', 2004 Nov, 53(11): 1617–1623, PMID 15479682.
74 Vissiennon, C. et al., 'Calcium antagonistic effects of ethanol myrrh extract in inflamed smooth muscle preparations', Präsentation anlässlich des Phytotherapiekongresses, 2013, *Phytotherapie im Spannungsfeld zwischen Forschung und Praxis*, March 8–10, Leipzig.
75 Langhorst, J. et al., 'Randomised clinical trial: a herbal preparation of myrrh, chamomile and coffee charcoal compared with mesalazine in maintaining remission in ulcerative colitis – a double-blind, double-dummy study', *Aliment Pharmacol Ther.* 4 July 2013.
76 Richert, Jan, *Colitis ulcerosa – Medikamente und Therapien bei der chronisch entzündlichen Darmerkrankung (CED) – mit einem Blick auf Neuentdeckungen und Alternativmedizin*, Epubli, Berlin, 2014, ISBN 978-3844282054.
77 Boller u. Sichrowski, 'Linderung der Entzündungserscheinungen bei Colitis ulcerosa durch lokale

Anwendung der Lakrize', Weiss, R.E., *Lehrbuch der Phytotherapie*, 6th edition, Hippokrates p. 151, ISBN: 3-7773-0675-4.
78 Jehle, E.C. et al., 'Kolonkarzinom, Rektumkarzinom, Analkarzinom' (PDF 1.2 MB) August 2003 ISSN 1438-8979 p. 1.
79 Krebs in Deutschland. Gesellschaft der empidemiologischen Krebsregister in Deutschland (GEKID) und Zentrum für Krebsregisterdaten.
80 Botteri, E. et al., 'Smoking and colorectal cancer, a meta-analysis', *Jama* 300, 2008, 276–278 PMID 19088354 (PDF).
81 Kono, S., 'Obesity, weight gain and risk of colon adenomas in Japanese men', *Jpn J cancer Res* 90, 1999 801–811, PMID 10543250.
82 Lee, K.J. et al., 'Physical activity and risk of colorectal cancer in Japanese men and women, the Japan Public Health Center-based prospective study', *Cancer Causes Control* 18, 2007, 199–209, PMID 17206529.
83 Neugut, A.I. et al., 'Obesity and colorectal adenomatous polyps', *J Natl Cancer Inst* 83, 1991 359–361 PMID 1995919.
84 Herold, Gerd, *Innere Medizin: eine vorlesungsorientierte Darstellung*, 2012, Herold, Köln 2012 ISBN: 978-3-9814660-1-0.
85 EPIC-Symposium 25 Jan 2007, 'Was schützt vor Krebs und Diabetes?', *MMW-Fortschr. Med.* No. 24/2007, 149. Jg., S. 16.
86 Scheloski, S., 'Weniger Darmkrebs durch mehr Ballaststoff', *DlfE-Pressemitteilung* 2/2003, com 3 May 2003.
87 Weisburger et al., 'Bile acids, but not neutral sterols, are tumor promoters in the colon in man and rodents, *Environ Health Perspect* 50 (1983) 101–107.
88 Lapré, J.A. et al., 'Dietary modulation of colon cancer risk: the roles of fat, fiber and calcium', *Trends Food Sci Technol* 3 (1992) 320–324.
89 Scheppach, W. et al., *Present knowledge in nutrition*, 6th ed., Nutrition Foundation, Washington 1990, pp. 80–87.
90 Koch, T.C. et al., 'Prevention of colon carcinogenesis by apple juice in vivo: impact of juice constituents and obesity', *Mol Nutr Food Res* 53510–511, PMID 20371763.
91 Fähndrich, C., 'Wirkung von Apfelsaft auf die Kolonkarzinogenese und deren Modulation durch Wachstumsfaktoren im Tierexperiment', Dissertation Tierärztliche Hochschule Hannover, 2005.

92 Offermann, S. et al., 'β-Carotin erhöht bei Rauchern und Trinkern das Darmkrebsrisiko', *Bild der Wissenschaft* (Online) vom 21.5.2003.
93 Watzerl, B. et al., *Bioaktive Substanzen in Lebensmitteln*, Hippokrates-Verlag Stuttgart, 1995, s.34 ISBN 3-7773-1115-4.
94 Bircher, A. et al., *Ganz besonders vor Krebs schützende Nahrungsmittel. Handbuch für Frischkost, Rohkost und Früchtespeisen*, Edition Bircher-Benner, Braunwald, 2014, pp. 22–24 ISBN 9 782979072232.
95 Lee, K.J. et al., 'Physical activity and risk of colorectal cancer in Japanese men and women, the Japan Public Health Center-based prospective study', *Cancer Causes Control* 18, 2007, 199–209, PMID 17206529.
96 Neugut, A.I. et al., 'Obesity and colorectal adenomatous polyps', *J Natl Cancer Inst* 83, 1991 359–361 PMID 1995919.
97 Galati, P.C. et al., 'Microbiological profile and nutritional quality of raw foods for neutropenic patients under hospital care, *Rev Bras Hematol Hemoter* 2013, 35(2) 94–98.
98 Branda, R.F. et al., 'Diet modulates the toxicity of cancer chemotherapy in rats', *J Lab Clin Med* 2002 Nov 140(5): 358–368 PMID12434138.
99 Conklin, K.A., 'Dietary antioxidants during cancer chemotherapy: impact on chemotherapeutic effectiveness and development of side effects', *Nutr Cancer* 2000, 37(1) 1–18.
100 Steven, J. et al., 'The benefit of the neurtopenic diet: fact or fiction?', *Oncologist* May 2011, 16(5): 704–707.
101 Bircher-Benner, M., *Ordnungsgesetze des Lebens*, Edition Bircher-Benner, Braunwald, 2014 p. 99.
102 Hoffmann, F.L., *Cancer and diet*, The Williams & Wilkins Company, Baltimore, 1937.
103 Van Vijck, R. et al., Utrecht University, 'An Introduction to Human Biophoton Emission', *Forsch Komplementärmed Klass Naturheilkd*, 1005,12, 77–83.
104 Bischof, M., *Biophotonen: das Licht in unseren Zellen*, ISBN 3-86150-095-7.
105 Popp, F.A., *Biologie des Lichtes, Grundlagen der ultraschwachen Zellstrahlung*, Verlag Paul Arex, ISBN: 3-489-61734-7.
106 Popp, F.A., *Unsere Lebensmittel in neuer Sicht*, ISBN 3-596-11459-4.

107 Gurwitsch, A.G., *Das Problem der Zellteilung*, Springer-Verlag, Berlin, 1926, *Die mitogenetische Zellstrahlung*, Springer-Verlag, Berlin 1932, and Arch. f. Mikr. Anat. und Entwicklungsmech, volumes 51, 52, 100, 101, 104.

108 Bircher-Benner, M.O., *Grundzüge der Ernährungstherapie auf Grund der Energie-Spannung der Nahrung*, Verlag Otto Salle, Berlin, 1905 and 1906.

109 Bircher-Benner, M.O., *Der zweite Hauptsatz der Energetik und die Ernährung*, Zschr der Wendepunkt, Wendepunktverlag, Zürich, 1936, Vom Wesen und der Organisation der Nahrungsenergie und über die Anwendung des zweiten Hauptsatzes der Energielehre auf den Nährwert und die Nahrungswirkung. Kleine Hippokratesbücherei Band 8 Hippokrates-Verlag Stuttgart und Leipzig 1936.

110 Pischinger, A., *Das System der Grundregulation. Grundlagen für eine ganzheitsbiologische Theorie der Medizin*, Haug-Verlag, Heidelberg, 1990, Seiten 13, 19, 78–82 8, expanded edition, ISBN 3 7760-1183-1.

111 Prigogine, I. et al., *Dialog mit der Natur*, Piper-Verlag München, ISBN 3-492-11191-5.

Index

6-Mercaptopurin	37, 41	Anxiety	36
		Apoptosis	30, 35, 36
Acetic acid	13	Appendicitis	25
Aching limbs	31	Appendix	11, 12
Acne	31	Appetite	19, 36
Acne rosacea	37	Apple diet week	38, 52
Actinobacteria	23	Arginin	10
Activation of the pancreatic enzymes	10	Arrhythmia	33
Adenocarcinoma of the large intestine	43	Arteriosclerosis	22
Adenocarcinoma of the oesophagus	15	Arthritis in Crohn's disease and colitis ulcerosa	36, 40
Adenoma of the stomach	18	Asthma bronchiale	33
Adrenal hormones	10	Atrophic gastritis	17
Adrenaline	10	Autoimmune disease	30
Aerobes	12	Autonomous nervous system	13
Aerophagia	26	Avenin A, E, F	29
AIDS	24	Azathioprine	37, 41
Albumin allergy	34		
Alcohol	9, 16, 17, 20, 26, 29, 33	Bacterial miscolonization of the intestine	32
α-cells of the pancreas	10	Bacterial miscolonization of the small intestine	33
α-defensin	35		
Alkaline intestinal milieu	13	Bacterial miscolonization of the stomach	18
Allergic immune reaction	11, 21		
Alzheimer's disease	22	Bacterial settlement of the intestine	12
Amines	13	Bacteroides	12, 13, 36
Amino acid spectrum of the food	9	Bakers' asthma	29
Amoebas	23	Barrett cancer	15
Amylase	8	Barrett syndrome	15, 16
Amylase inhibitors IAM1, CMb	29	Basic substance, matrix	22
Anaemia	19, 26, 28, 36, 41	Belching	15, 17
		Beta carotene	44
Anaerobic, obligate, facultative	12, 23	β-cells of the pancreas	10
Animal-based food	18, 20	β-defensin	35
Animal-based protein and fat	13	Bifidus bacteria	12, 23, 36
Anserines (Potentilla anserina)	42	Bile	10
Anthrocyane	25	Bile acids, primary, secondary	10, 11
Antibiotically active food	25	Biogeneous amines	50
Antibiotic damage	26, 28, 32	Biological availability of food	51
Antioxydative effect of food	48	Biological information	49
Antrum pylori	9	Biologically-organic quality	51
Anus	12		

Biopsy of the mucosa of the small intestine	30
Black tea, green tea	20
Bland Healing Diet	58
Bleeding from the intestine	39, 43
Bloatedness	15, 17
Blood pressure drip	33
Blood sugar test	31
Blood type A and stomach cancer risk	18
Bloody-slimy diarrhoea	40
Body compress	31
Bosweila serrata	41
Bottle-fed children	23
Branched-chained fatty acids	13, 36
Bread, fresh	26
Breastfeeding	23
Budesonide	37, 41
Butter	51
Buttermilk diet	25, 53
Butyric acid	13, 23, 44
Cabbage	26
Caecum	11
Calcium	31
Calories	48
Cancer of the large intestine	40, **43**
Cancer of the large intestine, prevention	43
Cancer of the large intestine, therapy, prognosis	44, 45
Cancer protection of the food	13
Cancer risk from colitis ulcerosa	40
Candida albicans	24, 29, 36, 39
Candidose	24, 29, 36, 39
Carbon dioxide gas	13, 23
Carcinogenic fats	51
Carcinoma of the small intestine	37
Cardia	8
Carotenoids	49
Casein	50
Casein allergy	34
CD4+ helper cells	30
Cereal dishes, recipes	65, **84**
Cereal gel	56
Chamomile enema	27, 52
Chaos principle of physics	48
Cheese	16, 24, 26, 31, 33, 34, 50, 51
Chlorophyll-A-molecules	47

Choanes	8
Chocolate	26, 32, 33, 50, 51, 58, 60
Cholangitis, primary sclerosing, ascending	40
Cholecystokinin	10, **14**
Chromosome 8 with only 3 alleles	35
Chylomicrons	10
Chymotrypsin	10
Chymus	11
Circulation impairmen	8
Civilisation diseases	48
Clostridia	12, 23, 36
Clostridium difficile	24
Cobalamin	11
Cobblestone relief	37
Coecal colitis	40
Coeliac disease	**28**, 57
Coenzyme Q10	38
Coffee	9, 16, 19, 20, 26
Coherence	47
Coherence principle of Prigogine	48
Colitis	17, 21
Colitis, infectious	22
Colitis ulcerosa	**39**, 44
Colitis ulcerosa, dietetic therapy of the cause	42
Colitis ulcerosa, surgical treatment	41
Colon	**11**
Colon Carcinoma	**43**
Colon carcinoma, early recognition	44
Colon carcinoma, genetic peculiarities	44
Colon carcinoma, prevention	43
Colon carcinoma, therapy, prognosis	44, 45
Colon irritabile	27
Colonisation resistance	23
Combustion heat (calories)	48
Commiphora myrrha	41
Conjugated bile acids	11
Constipation	**22**, 59
Constipation, tendency to, permanent diet	59
Cooking, value loss	19, 71
Cortisol	10, 37, 41
Cow milk, industrial processing	50
Cream	27, 34, 50, 51
Cress	25, 49
Crohn's disease	**34**, 44
Crohn's disease, general symptoms	36

Crohn's disease, therapy	37		Escherichia coli	12, 23
Cyclosporine	41		Escherichia coli Nissle 1917	40, 41
Cystic fibrosis	20		Eubacteria	12, 23, 36
			Exhaustion crises	40
Degeneration	7, 26, 31, 48		Exocirne pancreas	20
Degraded food	26		Expectant tension and diarrhoea	22
δ-cells of the pancreas	10		Explosive discharges	24
Depression	21, 32			
Desoxycholic acid	44		Fatigue after a meal	11
Desserts, recipes	90		Fats	51
Detoxifying	22		Fatty acids, saturated, unsaturated	9, 10, 30
Detoxing	22		Fatty acids, short-chained and	
Diabetes mellitus	22, 29		protection from cancer	13
Diaminoxydase	33		Fatty liver	17
Diaphragmal hernia	15		Fatty stool, floating stool	20
Diarrhoea	22, 52, 53		Fear of examinations and diarrhoea	28
Diarrhoea, summer catarrh, acute, diet	52		Fermentation	13, 15, 17, 21, 23, 28, 48
Digestion dyspepsia	17			
Digestion problems	17		Ferroportin	35
Digestive enzymes of the pancreas	9		Fibre	13, 23, 44
Dissipative system according			Firmicutes	13, 23
to Prigogine	48		Fish	44
Diverticula, diverticulitis, diverticulosis	**42**		Fistula formation	37, 43
DNA, deoxyribonucleic acid	47		Flatulence tea	27, 52, 62, 98
Dressings, recipes	66		Flatulence, meteorism	24, **26**
Ductus choledochus	10		Flavour enhancer	32
Ductus pancreaticus	9		Folic acid	30, 32
Duodenal ulcer	18, **21**		Food allergy	33, 34
Duodenum	9		Food economy according	
Dysbiose s. bacterial miscolonization	34, 36		to Bircher-Benner	48, 58
Dysmenorrhoe	33		Food effect on the digestion, summary	98
			Food energy, two kinds	47
Eggs	16, 24, 26, 50		Food sensitivity	33, 34
Electrolyte loss	12		Food that protects from cancer	18, 19, 44
Emptying of the stomach	9, 17, 27		Foreign body feeling	16
Endobrachyal oesophagus	15		Frankincense (Bosweila serrata)	41
Endocrine pancreas	10		Free fatty acids	9, 10
Energetic value of food	48		Fresh juice diet	26, 52, **53**
Energy, ordered, chaotic	47		Fresh juices and gruel diet	53, 62
Enteritis	**21**		Fructose intolerance, congenital,	
Enteritis regionalis	35		acquired	24, **32**, 38
Entero bacteria	12		Fruit and cancer protection	18, 44
Enterococci	12, 23		Fruits, secondary vegetable	
Enterocytes	35, 36		substances, effect	49
Enterohepatic circulation	**11**, 37		Fundus of the stomach	9
Episcleritis	40		Fungus infestation and intestine	24
Eradication of Helicobacter pylori	18		Fusobacteria	12, 23, 36
Erectile dysfunction	41			
Erythema nodosum	36, 40		Galactose	31

Gall bladder, discharge	10, 14	Homogenisation of milk	34, 50
Gall problems	11, 17, 20	Hordenin	29
Gall stones	20	Hormonal regulation of digestion	**13**
Ganglia	13	Hospitalism	24
Ganglion coeliacum	13, 39	Hot drinks and oesophagus carcinoma	16
Gas formation, toxic (s. intestinal rot)	36	Hot spices	26, 51, 58
Gastric acid regulation	9, 18	Hydrocolon therapy	27
Gastric ulcer	18	Hydrogen gas	13, 31
Gastrin	9, **14**	Hydrogen sulphur gases	36, 49
Gastritis	**17**, 18	Hydrogen superoxide	19
Gene CARD15/NOD2-defect	35		
General physical treatments	102	Ig-antibodies	11, 38
Genetic mutation and colon carcinoma	43	IgG 4 food allergy test	34, 38
		Ileitis terminalis	34
GIP (glucose-dependant insulinotropic peptide) Gliadin C-C antigen α, β, ω	9, **14**	Ileum	**11**
		Ileus	37, 44
Gliadin	29	Immune defence	12
Gliadin-antibodies	30	Immune system of the intestine	**12**, 13, 29
Glucagon	10	Immunomodulating food	49
Glucose	10	Impotence	41
Glue protein	29	Impulse to defecate	12
Glutamine	29, 30	Indole	13
Glutathione	38	Infant formula food	50
Gluten	29	Inflammation-inhibition, food for	98
Gluten allergy search tests	29	Information, storage, transfer	48
Gluten-sensitive enteropathy	29	Inhibited growth	30
Gluten sensitivity	29	Insulin	10
Glycerine	9, 10	Insulin release	14
Goblet cells	9	Interferon γ	30
		Interleukin 1 and 6	30
H_2-blocker	15	Intestinal catarrh	**21**
H_2-breathing test	32	Intestinal flora	**12**, 42
Haemorrhoids	11, 12, 24	Intestinal infantilism	28
Headache	21, 31, 32, 33	Intestinal mucosa barrier	29
Healing earth	25, 27	Intestinal peristalsis	21
Heartburn	62	Intestinal polyp	40, 43, 44
Heart pain	9	Intestinal rot	24
Heat, inner	36	Intrinsic factor	11, 26
Helicobacter pylori	18	Iron deficiency	18, 31, 35, 36, 38
Hepcidin	35		
Herter-Heubner's disease	**28**	Irritable bowel syndrome	**27**, 32
Hiatus hernia	15	Irritated hunger	8, 17
Histamine	14, 15	Islet cells of the pancreas	10, 14
Histamine intolerance	**33**	Isobutyric acid	36
Histamine level	33	Isovalerian acid	36
Histamine N-methyl transferase	33		
Histocompability antigens HLA-I, DR, DQ	30	Jaundice, epidemic	17
		Jejunum	**10**
Homoeopathic treatment	39	Juices diet, fresh juice diet	53, 61

Killer cells, natural	49
Kousa days	53
Lactase	31
Lactic acid, lactate	23, 50
Lactobacilli	12, 23
Lactose-free diet	31
Lactose intolerance, congenital, acquired	31
Lactose mal-digestion	31
Lactulose	23
Lamblia	23
Laser light storage, rhythmic	47, 48
Laser threshold	47
Law of entropy	48
Laxatives	23
LCT-genotype	32
Lecithin	42
Lienteria	24
Light accumulation according to Bircher-Benner Lipase	48
Lipids	10
Lipo proteins	10
Liquorice	42
Lithocholic acid	44
Liver	18, 22
Low-acid stomach	17
Lymph cell nests of the intestine	12
Lymphocytes	12
Lymphoma	29
Lymph system of the intestine	11
Machine preparation forms of food	50
Macrophages (scavenger cells)	49
Magnesium	31, 41
Malabsorption	20, 37, 38
Matrix, basic substance of the connective tissue	22
Meat	44
Menstrual problems	33
Mental traumas	22, 23, 36
Menus by various consistency forms	94
Mercaptan	36
Mesazalin	41
Metabolic fault	51
Meteorism	26
Methane gas	13, 23
Methotrexate	37, 41
Methylthioxal	19

Methyl xanthine	19
Migraine	22, 33
Milk protein allergy	28, 33, 34
Milk types, recipes	70
Miscolonization of the intestine	21, 23, 28, 29, 32, 36
Miscolonization of the small intestine	24
Miscolonization of the stomach	18, 21
Mitochondria	10, 38
Mitochondrial infusion therapy	38
Monocytes	49
Motilin	**14**
Movement, daily, cancer protection from	16, 18, 23
Mucosa barrier	35, 36, 42
Mueslis	63
Mutaflor	40
Mycobacterium avium paratuberculosis antibodies	36
Myrrh	41
Nausea	32
Nervousness	31
Neural therapy	25, 39, 43
Neurogenic amines	36
NFKB-transcription factor	39
Nicotine abuse (smoking)	9, 20, 26
Nitrite	18
Nitrogen gases	24
Non-Hodgkin lymphoma	29
Nosocomial infection	24
Obesity	17, 20
Obesity and gastritis	17
Obesity and intestinal flora	12
Obesity intestinal flora as partial cause	13
Obesity, intestinal flora as partial cause	13
Oesophageal cancer (carcinoma)	**16**
Oesophagus hernia	15
Olive oil, heat-ability	51, 57, 59
Omeprazole	15
Oral cancer	8
Order therapy and cancer	43, 13
Organically biological quality	51
Osteopenia	30
Osteoporosis	37, 38, 40
Over-acidification of the stomach	9, 17, 54
Oxalate kidney stones	37

117

p-ANCA	35	Quark	24, 31, 33, 50
Pancreas	20		
Pancreas, diseases of the	20	Ranitidine	15
Pancreas insufficiency, exocrinous, endocrinous	20	Raw apple diet	49
		Raw food diet	16, 20, 24
Pancreatic cancer	20	Raw food diet, energetic information effect	48
Pancreatitis	20		
Parasympathicus	13	Raw food therapy and wound healing	45
Parietal cells	9	Raw food therapy, supporting cancer treatment	18, 20
Pepsin	9		
Perforation of the intestine (Peritonitis)	40	Recipes	61
		Rectum	11, 12
Peristalsis	8, 10, 11, 13, 14, 21	Reflux	9, **15**, 32
		Reflux esophagitis	15
Peritonitis	43	Rhematic disease and intestinal dysbiose	36
Phosphorus	31		
Photon storage, intra-cellular	47, 48	Rhythmic increase, laser principle	48
Photosynthesis	47	Roasted substances, roasting, barbecuing, frying	9, 19, 20, 26
Picking salt	51		
Plant coal	21	Rosaburia	23
Plant milk	32	Rosacea	37
Plexus solaris	13	Rot dyspepsia s. interstinal rot	24
Polyps	43, 44	Ruminococci	12, 23, 36
Polyps in Colitis ulcerosa	39, 40		
Portal vein system	10, 11, 12	Sacroileitis at Colitis ulcerosa	40
Potassium	15, 52	Salad dressings	66
Potato dishes	82	Salazosulfapyridin	37
Potato juice, raw	16, 27	Salivary glands	8
Prednisone	37, 39, 41, 42	Salt loss	12
Preserves food, preservatives	40, 64	Salt, use, daily amount	51
Priessnitz compress	26, 52	Sandwiches, recipes	89
Problems swallowing	15, 16	Sauces	87
Procaine base infusion	38	Sclerosing, chronic enteritis	35
Proctitis	24	Sea salt	51, 58
Proline	29	Secalin	29
Propionic acid	13	Secondary plant substances	38, 49
Propulsion movement	12	Second principle of thermo dynamics	48
Protective healing diet	59	Secretin	9, 10, **14**
Protein containing nutrients	99	Selenium	31, 38, 41
Proteins, biological value	50	Senna	23
Proteobacteria	23	Sense of taste	8, 58
Proteoglycans	22	Sensitivity to cold	27
Protozoa	13	Sensitivity to weather	21
Pseudomembranose enterocolitis	24	Serotonin	32
Pureed diet	56	Short-chained fatty acids	13, 24
Putrefaction intestinal	23, 24, 28, 48	Sigma	11
Pylorus of the stomach	9	Sleeplessness	13
Pyoderma gangraenosum	36	Slime layer of the small intestine	10
		Slow-waves	49

Smoking	9, 18, 19, 20, 26	Toxic megacolon	37, 40
Sodium bicarbonate	9, 10, 15	Transglutaminase	29, 30
Sodium loss	41	Trypsin	10
Sodium-potassium ATPase	15	Tryptophan	32
Solar plexus	13	Tuberculosis, reactivation	38
Somatomedin	10	Tumour necrosis factor α	30, 37, 41
Somatostatin	14		
Soups	71	UHT treatment of milk	34
Sour intestinal milieu	12, 23	Ulcus duodeni	18, 21
Sour milk diet	24, 38, **50**	Ulcus gastrici	18
Spondylitis ankylosans at		Ultra-weak light radiation (Gurwitsch)	47
Colitis ulcerosa	40	Unrest, inner	31
Sprue, domestic, tropical	29	Uveitis	37, 40
Squamous cell carcinoma of			
the oesophagus	16	Vagus nerve	8, 10, **13**
Starch	8, 10, 50	Vegan diet	38
Starch-containing nutrients	10	Vegetable margarine, effect	51
Stomach cancer	18	Vegetable salad, cooked, recipes	65
Stool incontinence	41	Vegetables, recipes	74
Stool mass	11, 12	Vegetative nervous system	9, 13, 39, 51
Strawberry diet day	52	Vertigo	31
Streptococci	23	Vital substances	21, 30, 48
Stress	9, 10, 13, 29	Vitamin A	25, 30, 49
Stress symptoms	36	Vitamin B	30
Succus liquiriziae	42	Vitamin B_2	21
Sugar	20, 25, 44	Vitamin B_6	33
Sugar-containing foods	50	Vitamin B_{12}	11, 21, 26, 36, 38
Sulfonamides	26		
Sunlight, information from	47, 48, 49	Vitamin C	18, 38, 49
Surface of the small intestine	10	Vitamin deficiency	26
Susceptibility to infection	31	Vitamin E	30
Swallowing	8, 15	Vitamin K	21
Sweating	31	Vitamins	31
Symbiosis control	38		
Sympathetic trunk	43	Wheat gel Dr. Kousa	56, 62, 98
Sympathicus	13, 36	White flour dishes	43, 44
		Wholemeal cereal, wholemeal and	
Table salt	26, 51	cancer protection	44
Tables for gastrointestinal patients	42	Worm infestation of the intestine	23
Tachycardia	36, 40	Wound healing, effect of	
Tea (health teas)	52, 62	raw food therapy	45
Thermodynamic balance	48		
Thiols	13	Yang	13
TIA transient ischaemic attack	15	Yin	13
Tights junctions	11, 35	Yoghurt	25, 27, 33, 50
Tissue transglutaminase	30		
TNF α-blockers	37, 41	Zinc	31, 32, 38, 41
Tonsils	12		
Tormentilla	42		

CENTRE FOR SCIENTIFIC NATURAL MEDICINE

CENTER FOR SCIENTIFIC NATURAL MEDICINE
BIRCHER-BENNER
BRAUNWALD

People come to the Bircher-Benner Medical Centre from a large number of countries in search of healing.

Here, you will be valued as a unique person, listened to and understood. Here, humanity and dignity are important and the medicine is a noble undertaking.

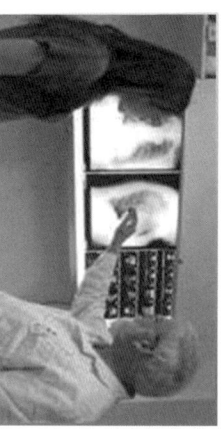

The search for the true causes of diseases is central to our work, as is the inclusion of your self-curative powers in the process of healing.

Indications: any internal diseases, migraine, tinnitus, neuralgia and other pain conditions, fibromyalgia, arthritis and arthrosis, collagenoses, liver, gallbladder and gastrointestinal diseases, metabolic diseases and diabetes, cardiovascular diseases, kidney and prostate diseases, women's diseases, allergies, skin diseases, convalescence, fatigue, depression and anxiety, menopausal, hormonal and weight problems.

Centre for scientific natural medicine

Our fresh-vegetable diet will bring about a rapid change in your metabolism; natural regulative therapies take precedence where possible.

The atmosphere and the living tradition of the Bircher-Benner Centre, where novelty and modernity are combined with decades of experience, contribute to your healing.

The doctors and therapists will treat you personally and have all the facilities of a modern clinic at hand when needed.

The supplementation of traditional medicine by the regulative diagnosis and therapy of natural healing often permits a cure where the usual therapies have failed.

In the Medical Centre, you can relax and recover, and will experience the deep regeneration of your healing powers.

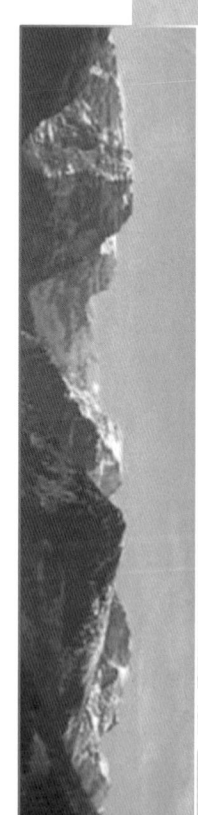

CENTRE BIRCHER-BENNER
CH-8784 Braunwald
Phone: +41 (0)21 801 60 04
Fax: +41 (0)55 643 16 93
info@bircher-benner.com
www.bircher-benner.com